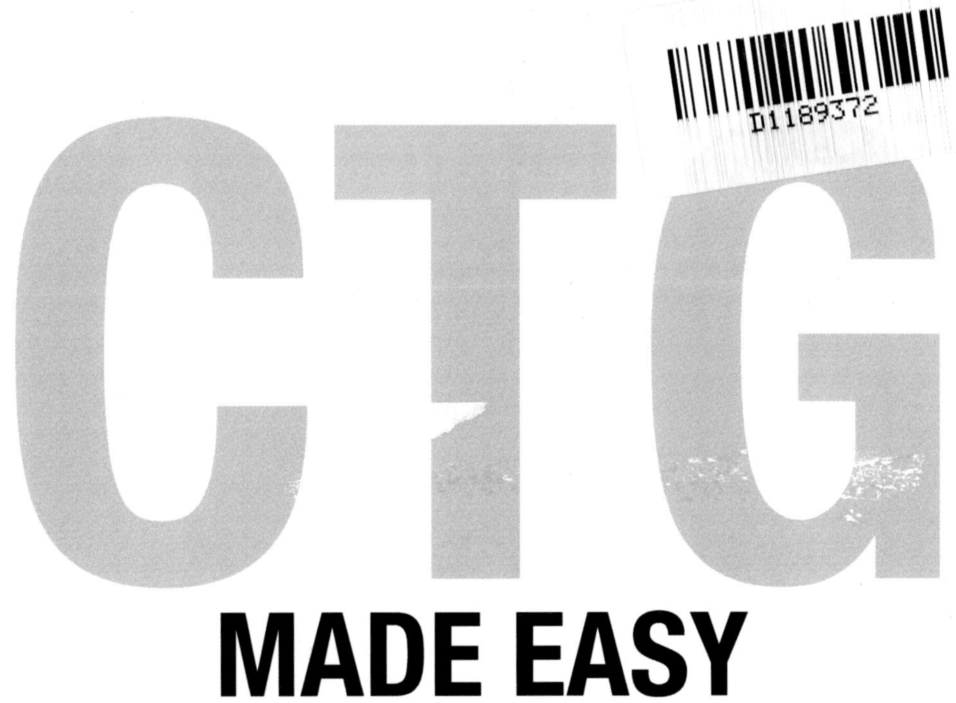

MADE EASY

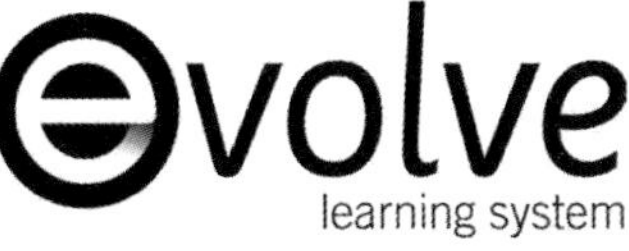

For Elsevier:
Commissioning Editor: Mairi McCubbin
Development Editor: Helen Leng
Project Manager: Sukanthi Sukumar
Designer: Charles Gray
Illustration Manager: Bruce Hogarth

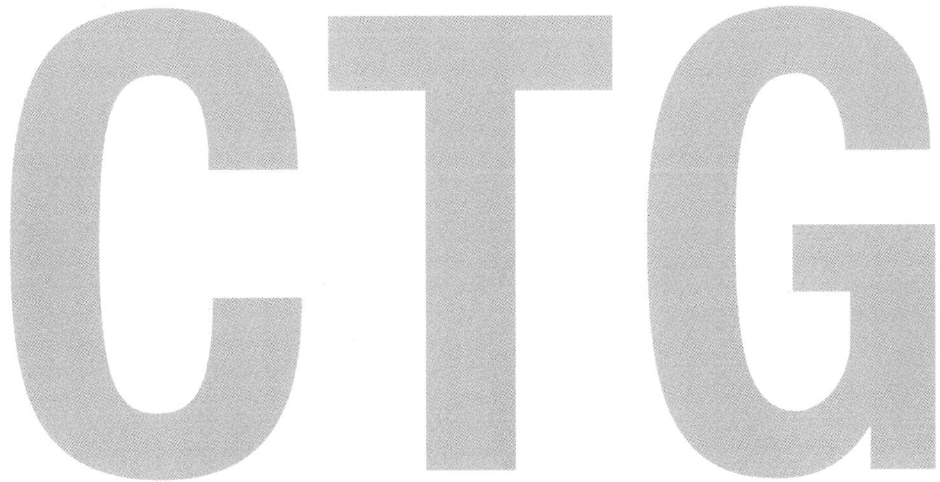

CTG MADE EASY

FOURTH EDITION

Susan M Gauge BSc(Hons) SRN SCM ADM ONC
Clinical Education Midwife, Delivery Suite, Birmingham Women's Healthcare NHS Trust, Birmingham, UK

With a contribution by
Andrew Symon MA(Hons) PhD RGN RM
Senior Lecturer, School of Nursing and Midwifery, University of Dundee, Dundee, UK

Foreword by
Tracey A Johnston MD FRCOG
Consultant in Maternal and Fetal Medicine, Birmingham Women's Hospital, Birmingham, UK

CHURCHILL LIVINGSTONE

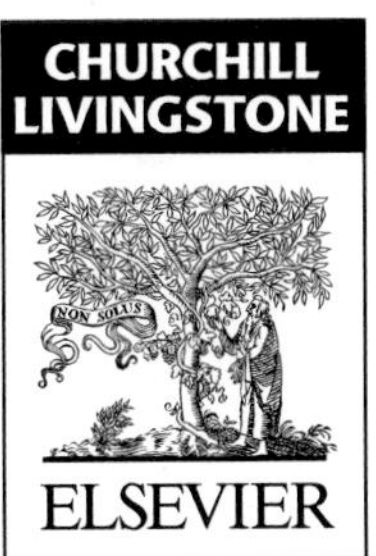

ELSEVIER

Edinburgh • London • New York • Oxford • Philadelphia • St Louis • Sydney • Toronto 2012

CHURCHILL
LIVINGSTONE
ELSEVIER

First edition 1992
Second edition 1999
Third edition 2005
Fourth edition 2012
Reprinted 2013 (twice), 2014, 2015

ISBN: 978-0-7020-5214-9

British Library Cataloguing in Publication Data
A catalogue record for this book is available from the British Library

Library of Congress Cataloging in Publication Data
A catalog record for this book is available from the Library of Congress

Notices
Knowledge and best practice in this field are constantly changing. As new research and experience broaden our understanding, changes in research methods, professional practices, or medical treatment may become necessary.

Practitioners and researchers must always rely on their own experience and knowledge in evaluating and using any information, methods, compounds, or experiments described herein. In using such information or methods they should be mindful of their own safety and the safety of others, including parties for whom they have a professional responsibility.

With respect to any drug or pharmaceutical products identified, readers are advised to check the most current information provided (i) on procedures featured or (ii) by the manufacturer of each product to be administered, to verify the recommended dose or formula, the method and duration of administration, and contraindications. It is the responsibility of practitioners, relying on their own experience and knowledge of their patients, to make diagnoses, to determine dosages and the best treatment for each individual patient, and to take all appropriate safety precautions.

To the fullest extent of the law, neither the publisher nor the authors, contributors, or editors, assume any liability for any injury and/or damage to persons or property as a matter of products liability, negligence or otherwise, or from any use or operation of any methods, products, instructions, or ideas contained in the material herein.

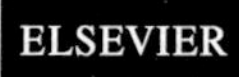

Printed in China

Contents

Online Contents

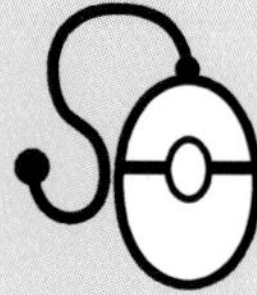

CASE STUDIES

Foreword

All of us involved in delivering intrapartum care have an obligation to the women and babies in our care, as well as to the institutions we work for and to ourselves, to be fully competent and confident in all aspects of intrapartum fetal monitoring. This is a basic requirement as an understanding of the mechanisms of labour. As Part 3 of this book highlights, errors in all aspects of fetal monitoring still occur, sometimes with profound consequences for the child and his/her family. Teaching and training are now more robust, and indeed form part of annual mandatory training, but fetal monitoring is still an area that causes many junior midwives and doctors some degree of anxiety. Most practitioners will consult a text to refresh and improve their knowledge, and this book does exactly what it says on the cover – makes CTG interpretation easy!

A basic knowledge of the physiology of fetal heart rate control is essential. It aids understanding of the changes seen in fetal monitoring and contextualises the changes taking place in the fetal circulatory system. The section on intermittent auscultation is particularly welcome, as some midwives feel they have lost their skills secondary to the reliance on electronic fetal monitoring that has predominated intrapartum care until recently, and many doctors have never learned the skill. This text gives a clear, evidence-based approach to all aspects of intrapartum fetal monitoring which is easy to read and understand. Part 4 then allows readers to put what they have learned into practice with the wide range of cases and scenarios. No matter what level of expertise exists, whether learning the skill of intrapartum fetal monitoring for the first time or refreshing existing knowledge, this text will benefit all practitioners, and in turn, the women and children we care for.

Tracey A Johnston MD FRCOG
Consultant in Maternal and Fetal Medicine
Birmingham Women's Hospital

Preface

Fetal heart rate monitoring during labour has become an accepted means of assessing the well-being of a baby. However, in order for the resulting data to be of value it is vital that midwives, obstetricians and students have a knowledge of the methods of fetal heart rate monitoring available, the physiology of fetal heart rate abnormalities, the recommended terminology that should be used when interpreting data (National Collaborating Centre for Women's and Children's Health 2007) and the appropriate management of such abnormalities.

It is important that women have a choice in the method of fetal heart rate monitoring during labour. Professionals must be able to give an explanation, based on available evidence, as to the risks and benefits of both intermittent auscultation and continuous electronic fetal heart rate monitoring, and these discussions are included in this text.

Developments in fetal heart rate monitoring are ongoing, particularly regarding the use of decision support software packages (Barber et al. 2010; Jameen et al. 2010). Whilst we aim to provide women with as normal experience as possible, electronic fetal heart rate monitoring is recommended for high-risk women in labour and the technology is becoming more complicated and, in some instances, more invasive. Professionals involved in the care of women in labour should be aware of these developments and the effects they may have on intrapartum care.

The information within this book will hopefully inform practitioners and motivate them to seek out results of ongoing and future research for the benefit of women within their care.

A number of texts are already in existence which describe in detail fetal physiology and monitoring techniques. It is not intended to cover the same ground in this book, but to complement them by providing a basic grounding in the physiology of fetal heart rate monitoring, the main focus being the initiation of discussions relating to the interpretation of cardiotocographs (CTGs). It is hoped that this will be achieved by providing a series of examples of CTGs produced during labour.

This book is aimed at all midwives, midwifery students, obstetricians and medical students and anyone with an interest in fetal heart rate monitoring. It is hoped that it will go some way towards increasing knowledge, confidence and competence and thereby maintaining safety for the women and babies we care for.

For those not familiar with the origin of the book, the idea of a case-study approach to aid the interpretation of CTGs arose in 1986 as a result of the Teaching and Assessing in Clinical Practice course for midwives. A teaching package was produced containing a number of case histories, including a section on the CTG, followed by an analysis and description of the management instituted at the time. The package was used extensively in a number of delivery suites by midwives and doctors, initiating lively discussion. We know, from the comments of many doctors and midwives in the UK, that *CTG Made Easy* is used widely, arouses debate and aids learning. The book has an international readership and has been translated into German, Chinese and French.

In this, the fourth edition, we continue to follow the previous format, but with a number of revisions and additions. Part 1 includes wider discussions and reference to published evidence regarding available methods of fetal monitoring, with more information relating to intermittent auscultation. Assessing risk in labour is discussed as well as more recent developments in fetal monitoring practice.

Part 2 has been expanded to include more information regarding the physiological control of fetal heart rate and CTG abnormalities. Reference is made to national recommendations for the categorisation of CTGs (National Collaborating Centre for Women's and Children's Health 2007) and a proforma to aid consistency in interpretation (Draycott et al. 2008).

Part 3, Litigation and the CTG, with its use of legal case studies to illustrate important lessons, has been updated and gives an insight into the role of the CTG when allegations of clinical negligence are investigated.

The case studies section, Part 4, has been reviewed. The CTGs have been interpreted in line with recommendations from the National Institute for Health and Clinical Excellence (National Collaborating Centre for Women's and Children's Health 2007) and new CTGs have been added. Questions concerning the CTG are raised for consideration by the reader or group, with the opportunity to make notes. In addition, 20 new cases are available online to complement the book.

Part 5 introduces a number of ways to develop good-practice initiatives that can be adapted to suit the needs of any trust.

Your comments on any aspect of the book are welcome, particularly if you have any useful guides to good practice that could be included in future editions.

I hope you find the changes helpful and that they will inform your judgements and decision-making in practice.

The value of this book will be in the richness of discussions arising from the case studies presented. Highlighting good practice may lead to further developments and review of existing guidelines. The benefits of this will only add to what every mother and baby deserves – practice that is safe, of the highest standard and results in an emotionally satisfying experience.

Birmingham, 2011 Susan M Gauge

REFERENCES

Barber, V. S., Lean, K. A., & Shakeshaft, C. E. (2010). Computers and CTGs: where are we at? *British Journal of Midwifery, 18*, 644–649.

Draycott, T., Winter, C., & Crofts, J. (Eds.), (2008). London: RCOG Press.

Jameen, J., Cross, D., & Cairns, J. (2010). Cardiotocography and ST analysis (STAN): a retrospective review. *British Journal of Midwifery, 18*, 568–574.

National Collaborating Centre for Women's and Children's Health (2007). *Intrapartum care. Care of healthy women and their babies during childbirth.* London: RCOG. Clinical guideline.

ACKNOWLEDGEMENTS

I would like to thank all those who have assisted with the production of this book, especially midwives Annette Gough and Jenny Henry who were involved with the initial teaching package on which the book was based.

Special thanks go to Christine Henderson whose motivation and persistence were seminal in the development of the book and best wishes are extended to her in her retirement.

I will also take this opportunity to acknowledge the special contribution of all the midwives, doctors and ward clerks on delivery suite at Birmingham Women's Health Care Foundation NHS Trust and the women they care for, without whom this book would not be possible.

Assessing fetal well-being in labour

PART 1

INTRODUCTION

Continuous monitoring of the fetal heart rate during labour became a widespread practice during the 1970s and has remained an accepted technique for assessing fetal well-being. The rapidity of the technological advance and acceptance into practice without prior evidence of the benefits and risks to women is well recognised (Arulkumaran and Chua 1996; Blincoe 2005; Walsh 2008). It becomes increasingly difficult to reduce the use of technology once it has become an accepted practice and McAra-Couper et al. (2010) argue that the acceptance of technology leads to deskilling of practitioners and ultimately an increase in interventions.

The purpose of fetal heart rate monitoring in labour is to record the fetal heart rate and uterine contractions, identifying changes to the fetal heart rate that may be indicative of a developing fetal compromise. This information provides practitioners with the opportunity to initiate further investigations or expedite the birth of the baby as appropriate, in an attempt to reduce the rates of long-term neurological damage in babies and children.

One of the earliest and largest randomised controlled trials comparing continuous electronic fetal heart rate monitoring (CEFM) with intermittent auscultation (IA) to monitor the fetal heart rate in labour was reported by MacDonald et al. in 1985. They concluded that IA was as reliable as CEFM in detecting fetal hypoxia in low-risk women. Subsequent studies report a higher incidence of operative vaginal deliveries and caesarean section when CEFM is used and a higher incidence of neonatal seizures without long-term neurological sequalae when IA is the method of monitoring used (Thacker et al. 1995; Supplee and Vezeau 1996; Mongelli et al. 1997; National Institute for Health and Clinical Excellence (NICE) 2004; Alfirevic et al. 2006).

The National Sentinel Caesarean Section Audit Report (Royal College of Obstetricians and Gynaecologists 2001a) identified that the most frequently cited primary reason for performing a caesarean section was presumed fetal compromise. There is evidence to suggest that maternal morbidity and mortality can be adversely affected by caesarean section (NICE 2004) and, while maternal mortality rates continue to fall, there is a link between death rates and caesarean section (Hall 2001; Confidential Enquiry into Maternal and Child Health 2007). Any unnecessary procedure that may increase the risk of caesarean section, such as CEFM in a low-risk woman, would therefore best be avoided.

A more recent review of 12 randomised controlled trials found no evidence that perinatal mortality was reduced in either low- or high-risk women when CEFM was used in labour (Alfirevic et al. 2006), although both the National Collaborating Centre for Women's and Children's Health (NCCWCH) 2007; and the NHS Litigation Authority (NHS Litigation Authority 2009) advocate the use of CEFM when risk factors are identified in labour. Debates continue about the risk categories assigned to women (Devane et al. 2010) and the reliability of CEFM for all women in labour (Walsh et al. 2008).

In practice today, guidelines recommend that CEFM, whether by means of an abdominal transducer or fetal scalp electrode, should be restricted to women who are in a high-risk category for labour whilst IA should be the preferred method of monitoring the fetal heart rate for low-risk women in labour (NCCWCH 2007). Munro et al. (2002) found evidence that CEFM rates had reduced following publication of the National Sentinel Caesarean Section Audit report (Royal College of Obstetricians and Gynaecologists 2001a). More recently, Churchill and Francome (2009) report a continuing decrease in routine CEFM, which is now less common than was identified by NICE in 2004.

Women should be given choices regarding their care (Department of Health 2007) and have access to literature relating to fetal monitoring in labour (NCCWCH 2007) in order for them to make informed decisions (Werkmeister 2007). It is acknowledged that advocating choice may present challenges for professionals (Royal College of Obstetricians and Gynaecologists 2007) when balancing safety with the woman's chosen preferences; therefore all professionals involved in caring for women in labour must be aware of the most recent recommendations and evidence relating to fetal monitoring in order to inform women fully of the risks and benefits before obtaining informed consent. The Health Care Commission (2007) reported that almost one-third of women do not always feel involved in decisions about their care in labour, so there are still improvements to be made. Midwives in particular should ensure that their knowledge is current, not only because they are the main care providers and advocates for the vast majority of women, but also because they have a professional responsibility to do so (Nursing and Midwifery Council 2004, 2008).

Progress is being made towards less intervention for low-risk women in labour and the promotion of normality (Allan and Talbot 2008), including the methods used for fetal heart rate monitoring. Midwives are being encouraged by national guidelines (NCCWCH 2007) to use their traditional skills to be with women during labour and birth. However, there remains a duty of care for the women who fall into high-risk categories. For these women available evidence still recommends that fetal well-being in labour should be assessed by CEFM (NICE 2004). The optimum outcome for mother and baby relies heavily upon the interpretation of the resulting data in the form of the cardiotocograph (CTG).

While the primary aim of this book remains to encourage standardised interpretation of the CTG, it is important to include assessment of the fetal heart rate in labour by means of IA.

INTERMITTENT AUSCULTATION

For low-risk women, IA for the assessment of fetal well-being in labour should be offered and recommended by the professional involved in her care (NICE 2004). This may be by means of the Pinard stethoscope or a hand-held Doppler (NICE 2004). The latter may have the benefit of being more comfortable for the woman in allowing her to remain mobile or in water for labour and birth, while still allowing the midwife access to estimate the fetal heart rate reliably (Garcia et al. 1985; Mahomed et al. 1994; Mainstone 2004). Harrison (2004) discusses the instruments used for auscultation, concluding that the hand-held Doppler has advantages over the Pinard stethoscope; however later correspondence gives a differing point of view (Soltani and Shallow 2004). Blake (2008) maintains that the hand-held Doppler is the most versatile instrument for IA. There is little recent literature available comparing the efficacy and acceptability of the Pinard stethoscope with hand-held Dopplers; therefore it is prudent for midwives to retain skills to use both to provide women with choice during labour and birth and when one of the instruments may be unavailable.

Concerns have been expressed about the ability to detect variability by auscultation (Harrison 2004), although some midwives feel confident in their abilities to detect variations from normal, both baseline and periodic changes, when using a Pinard stethoscope (Association of Radical Midwives 2000).

Assessment of risk

Prior to commencement it is important that suitability for low-risk care in labour is identified following an accurate assessment of risk factors. Risk should be assessed at the onset of labour. Some women who were high-risk in the antenatal period, i.e. previous preterm birth, may be reassessed as low-risk in labour at term and be suitable for IA.

At the initial assessment of a woman in labour it is necessary to review the records made during the antenatal period, in both hand-held records and hospital case notes, in addition to documenting observations made during contact with the midwife. Note should be taken of:

- medical, surgical and obstetric history
- complications arising during the pregnancy
- estimated fetal growth using customised growth chart
- specific instructions from lead care professional regarding care in labour
- gestational age
- blood pressure, temperature and pulse rate
- pattern of fetal movements
- auscultated fetal heart rate
- colour of any liquor present
- uterine activity
- woman's choice regarding method of fetal heart rate monitoring.

Providing there are no pre-existing or pregnancy-related conditions or complications on initial assessment that may affect the progress of labour or oxygen supply to the fetus, and the woman agrees, IA should be the method of fetal heart rate monitoring offered and used.

Continual assessment

Risk factors can arise at any point during labour and vigilance is required in order to identify these and consider changing to CEFM. Midwives and obstetricians must remain alert to this throughout the labour. NCCWCH (2007) recommends commencing CEFM in the following instances:

- at the woman's request
- in the presence of meconium-stained liquor
- where there are concerns regarding the auscultated fetal heart rate, i.e. rate below 110 bpm, above 160 bpm, decelerations or rate persistently the same, which may be indicative of a reduction in variability
- when there is maternal pyrexia
- with fresh vaginal bleeding during labour
- with the use of oxytocin infusion for induction or augmentation of labour.

There may be occasions when deviations from the normal fetal heart rate are heard during auscultation. CEFM may be initiated in light of these findings but the subsequent CTG may well be classified as normal. This can provide reassurance for the midwife and woman and IA can be resumed. Care must be taken that intermittent CTG recordings in labour are not used routinely as a means of reassurance for midwives not confident in their practice (Altaf et al. 2006; Hindley et al. 2007), but for identified clinical need. If recurrent intermittent recordings are being made, risk assessment should be reviewed and CEFM considered.

Method of IA

The fetal heart rate should be auscultated at first contact in labour and at each subsequent contact during early labour (NCCWCH 2007). The maternal pulse rate should be assessed and recorded prior to auscultation. If there is any doubt about the rate of the fetal heart, the maternal pulse and fetal heart should be assessed simultaneously.

There is little evidence available to inform us of the optimum intervals and duration of IA during labour (Royal College of Obstetricians and Gynaecologists 2001b) but current recommendations state that, once labour is established, the fetal heart rate should be auscultated following a contraction for at least one full minute at the following intervals:

- at least every 15 minutes in the first stage
- at least every 5 minutes in the second stage (NCCWCH 2007).

The NHS Litigation Authority (2009) requires maternity services to demonstrate that practitioners comply with guidelines relating to the equipment that should be used for IA, when to auscultate the fetal heart, for how long, where this should be documented and when to palpate the maternal pulse rate.

Documentation

The rate of the fetal heart counted for 1 minute should be documented after each auscultation. When the maternal pulse rate has been counted at the same time this should also be recorded. Accurate documentation of the fetal heart rate is essential, preferably in chart form (see Good practice guide) as it is easier to identify progressive changes to the baseline rate: although this may still fall within the normal range, it may have altered significantly during the course of labour and require further action.

While there are still some issues relating to IA that would benefit from further research, such as frequency of auscultation and instrument of choice, it is recommended as a safe method of assessing fetal well-being in labour for low-risk women (NCCWCH 2007). There is evidence to suggest that practice is moving away from CEFM for all women (Munro et al. 2002; Churchill and Francome 2009) and, while it is excellent news that we are no longer totally reliant upon machines, it has to be remembered that the technology still has its place in clinical care. The important factor is having sufficient knowledge and experience to use it when required and confidence in IA where indicated.

CONTINUOUS ELECTRONIC FETAL HEART RATE MONITORING

CEFM involves the continual recording of the fetal heart rate and uterine activity by means of either external transducers placed on the abdomen or an internal scalp electrode attached to the fetal head with an abdominal transducer to record uterine activity. These are attached to a fetal heart rate monitor which prints out the CTG for interpretation.

Altaf et al. (2006) report on the risks and benefits that midwives attribute to CEFM which are reflected in prior and subsequent literature (Hindley et al. 2007). Some of the benefits attributed to CEFM are that a paper record is produced which allows a retrospective review of the fetal heart rate during labour and assists with the identification of developing abnormalities. This can also be used in clinical audit and for training purposes. If there has been an adverse outcome, the paper CTG is also relied upon when discussing the care with parents and for medicolegal purposes. For this reason CTGs must be kept for a minimum of 25 years (NCCWCH 2007). Ideally, the original CTG should remain in the case notes; if it is necessary to remove it for any reason, such as training or audit purposes, tracers in the case notes must indicate where the CTG can be found (NCCWCH 2007).

There are disadvantages to CEFM: the midwife's attention can be directed to the monitor instead of the woman, normal birth rates are significantly lower when CEFM is used (Alfirevic et al. 2006) and the rate of other interventions such as epidural analgesia and augmentation of labour with oxytocic drugs is increased (Munro et al. 2002; Alfirevic et al. 2006). Mobility of the woman is restricted although developments in telemetry (Boos et al. 1995; Phillips Health Care 2008; GE Healthcare 2010) which give a good-quality CTG and allow women to move around more freely, including using birth pools, can minimise this. In addition the interpretation of the CTG is subjective and has a high false-positive rate (Walsh 2008). Nelson et al. (1996) reported false-positive rates of 99.8% when predicting cerebral palsy from decelerative patterns on a CTG.

Reports from a confidential enquiry concentrating on intrapartum deaths highlighted suboptimal intrapartum care in 75.6% of cases, the most common criticism being the failure to recognise abnormalities occurring on the CTG (Confidential Enquiry into Stillbirths and Deaths in Infancy 1997). Another previous study concerned with obstetric litigation also highlighted failure to respond to CTG abnormalities as a problem (Ennis and Vincent 1990). This continues to be a clinical concern, as Nicholson and Saunders (2010) report over a third of negligence claims still feature misinterpretation of the CTG. The clinical value of CEFM is reliant upon the interpretation of the resultant data, the CTG. There are consistent reports from studies that demonstrate a poor rate of inter- and intraobserver agreement on the interpretation of CTGs (Ayres-de-Campos et al. 1999; Blix et al. 2003; Devane and Lalor 2005).

The technique is not without difficulties. It is reliant upon Doppler ultrasound via an abdominal transducer to detect the fetal heart, which itself has limitations. The Medicines and Healthcare products Regulatory Agency (2010) recommends that practitioners do not rely solely upon the CTG recording for the assessment of fetal well-being and are aware of limitations and possible artefacts. Certain factors will influence the strength of the signals detected:

- fetal activity
- maternal obesity
- maternal position
- maternal abdominal movements when coughing/vomiting/pushing in second stage.

The signals may not be strong enough to produce a good-quality CTG, leading to difficulty with accurate interpretation of the data. There have been reports of stillbirths occurring, despite a normal CTG (Medical Devices Agency 2002; Neilson et al. 2008; Medicines and Healthcare products Regulatory Agency 2010), attributed to the Doppler detecting a signal from maternal blood vessels in the absence of a fetal heart. It is recommended that the presence of the fetal heart is established by auscultation with either a Pinard stethoscope or hand-held Doppler prior to commencing a CTG (Medical Devices Agency 2002; NCCWCH 2007; Phillips Health Care 2009). If there is any doubt as to the rate of the fetal heart recording on the CTG during the labour, it is advisable to auscultate and write the counted rate on the CTG.

Despite improved technology there are still incidents reported when fetal monitors either halve or double the actual fetal heart rate (Phillips Health Care 2009), which can lead to inappropriate management, delayed or unnecessary interventions. Bhogal and Reinhard (2010) discuss the benefits of recording the maternal and fetal heart rates simultaneously with an abdominal maternal and fetal electrocardiogram (ECG) monitor to avoid possible confusion.

It is vital that the printed CTG is of good quality to ensure accurate interpretation of the data is possible. If this cannot be maintained externally, as a last resort a fetal scalp electrode can be applied to the baby's head. Women should be made aware at the commencement of CEFM that this is a possibility, particularly when difficulties are anticipated, such as obesity (Veerareddy et al. 2009). This can give a more accurate recording of the fetal heart rate but again is not without problems. There is potential for the maternal heart rate to be picked up in the absence of a fetal heart, the resulting printout being mistaken for fetal heart rate recording (Mainstone 2004). In order to apply the electrode the membranes must be ruptured and there will be a small wound on the baby's head: this increases the risk of infection and is contraindicated if there are known blood-clotting disorders or blood-borne infections such as human immunodeficiency virus (HIV) or hepatitis B.

Indications for CEFM

The clinical value of CEFM has been evaluated (Thacker et al. 2001; Alfirevic et al. 2006) and debated (Walsh 2008). Despite the lack of strong evidence to support the benefits of CEFM for all babies it is still the recommended method of monitoring the fetal heart rate for high-risk labours and births (NCCWCH 2007). A risk assessment should be completed at the onset of labour to identify high-risk women. Women's preferences for the method of fetal heart rate monitoring must also be sought. Some women may choose to have CEFM based on previous experiences and their wishes should be abided by.

Essentially a woman with any condition present that may adversely affect the oxygen transfer from mother to fetus will be high-risk. It is important to remember that, even though the antenatal period may have been without complications, there will be added stress to the fetus in labour from uterine contractions, which will further decrease oxygen transfer. Draycott et al. (2008) categorise risk factors into maternal, fetal and intrapartum problems.

Maternal problems

- medical conditions such as diabetes mellitus, renal and cardiac disease
- pregnancy-induced hypertension
- previous scar on uterus
- postterm pregnancy, over 42 weeks
- antepartum haemorrhage
- induced labour

Fetal problems

- intrauterine growth restriction
- oligohydramnios
- multiple pregnancy
- prematurity
- presence of meconium-stained liquor

Intrapartum problems

- auscultated fetal heart rate abnormality
- maternal pyrexia
- oxytocin augmentation
- fresh bleeding per vaginam
- epidural analgesia: a CTG should be performed for 30 minutes after initial commencement and after each bolus dose of 10 mL or more.

Note that this is not an exhaustive list.

Education and training

The CTG only becomes a valuable method of monitoring and assessing fetal well-being in labour if the professionals involved are confident in the use of the equipment, their skills in interpretation of the CTG and their knowledge of the correct management of fetal heart rate abnormalities. The high rates of inter- and intraobserver error in the interpretation of CTGs have been referred to earlier (Devane and Lalor 2005; Nicholson and Saunders 2010) and recent guidelines and training packages for fetal heart rate monitoring include standardised guides to fetal heart rate abnormalities and their recommended management (Beckley et al. 2000; Royal College of Obstetricians and Gynaecologists 2001b; NCCWCH 2007; Draycott et al. 2008).

Developing and maintaining expertise in the interpretation of CTGs requires regular training and updating (Royal College of Obstetricians and Gynaecologists 2001b; Nursing and Midwifery Council

2004, 2008; NCCWCH 2007; NHS Litigation Authority 2009). A study by Altaf et al. (2006) reported that midwives were satisfied with the available training yet they found that in practice there was a high rate of deviation from the evidence-based guidelines for both IA and CEFM and both doctors and midwives did not routinely document their opinions and care plans related to interpretation of CTGs. This is of concern, particularly for midwives who have a professional duty to maintain and develop their competence (Nursing and Midwifery Council 2004, 2008). In addition there are implications for the future as learners (student midwives, medical students and newly qualified midwives) tend to adopt the practices of their mentors, thus compounding potentially harmful practices (Armstrong 2010).

The development of clinical practice guidelines for fetal heart rate monitoring should have a multidisciplinary approach. They should be disseminated to all appropriate staff and be available within the clinical areas. Most often this will be by means of hospital intranet sites to which all staff should have easy access. Eccles et al. (2005) discuss the variable levels of success in incorporating guideline recommendations into clinical practice while Hollins Martin (2008) describes an approach to changing behaviour and implementing practice developments. Supervisors of midwives are ideally placed to ensure that midwives are knowledgeable about current practice guidelines.

Excellent communication must be maintained in order that all practitioners are made aware of current guidelines and regular multidisciplinary case note reviews or clinical discussions which include the CTG, interpretation and actions taken to provide useful learning opportunities. Audits of compliance with fetal monitoring guidelines should be regularly performed by midwives and doctors and the findings and recommendations fed back to all professionals by multidisciplinary presentations, notice board displays in the clinical area and via e-mail for staff who find difficulties in accessing training during the day.

Multiprofessional education and training reportedly has a positive impact on team working and therefore care of women (Ireland et al. 2008) and should be encouraged for training in interpretation of CTGs. It encourages understanding of roles and responsibilities and facilitates clear communication between professionals. Midwives and medical staff must have confidence in each other's clinical abilities in order to provide appropriate care for women in labour. Fraser and Blanas (2007) explore the impact of less experienced midwives calling doctors in to review CTGs on numerous occasions when there is no deterioration in the fetal heart rate and the increased anxiety this generates for the woman and the subsequent increase in interventions.

Training and updating in fetal heart rate monitoring should not be restricted to the interpretation of the CTG. Sessions should include information on the following:

- assessing risk at onset of labour
- guidelines for IA
- guidelines for CEFM
- equipment required for IA and CEFM and how to use it
- maintenance of equipment, including what to do if it is not working
- record keeping, documentation and storage of records
- findings from trust audits relating to fetal heart rate monitoring
- statistics relating to number of women monitored using IA and CEFM, normal birth, instrumental birth and caesarean section rates within the trust
- the normal fetal heart rate
- fetal heart rate abnormalities, aetiology and actions to be taken
- interpretation of CTGs using actual cases ensuring confidentiality is maintained
- fetal blood sampling, indications and interpretation of results.

Ideally this training would be incorporated into emergency skills drills training and attended on an annual basis (Draycott et al. 2008). All individual practitioners are responsible for ensuring that they maintain current knowledge and are able to use it in their clinical practice in order to provide safe care to women and babies.

ADJUNCTS TO CEFM FOR FETAL SURVEILLANCE

In addition to the CTG, further information is required in order to obtain objective information about the fetal condition in labour (Van Laar et al. 2008). Technological advances have been made, although some are poorly evaluated and few randomised controlled trials have been conducted. It is therefore not appropriate that they should be widespread in clinical practice. It is essential that further interventions should be thoroughly evaluated before being recommended routinely. The procedures are invasive and therefore have the potential to lead to other interventions and may not be acceptable to women in labour. All of the developments discussed are used in addition to CEFM and rely upon the accurate interpretation of the CTG.

Fetal blood sampling

This involves taking a sample of blood from the scalp of the fetus and measuring, primarily the pH and base deficit, estimating the acid-base balance and has been practised for many years (Saling and Schneider 1967). It is contraindicated in the presence of blood-borne infections such as HIV and hepatitis and clotting disorders (East et al. 2010) and also when the gestation is less than 34 weeks (NCCWCH 2007).

The procedure is invasive, uncomfortable and often painful for the woman and can be difficult to perform if the cervical os is less than 3 cm dilated. The sample must be free from contamination with amniotic fluid and air so that the acid-base balance can be estimated accurately. Staff must also be trained in the use of the equipment and guidelines for the management of fetal blood sampling must be current and disseminated to the professionals involved (NHS Litigation Authority 2009).

NICE (NCCWCH 2007) recommends the use of fetal blood sampling in the presence of a pathological CTG unless there is evidence of acute fetal compromise, such as a prolonged deceleration lasting 3 minutes or longer, when the baby should be delivered urgently.

Fetal blood sampling for lactate estimation has been investigated (East et al. 2010). The authors conclude that the technique is more likely to be successful than fetal blood sampling and results are more readily available. However, there is little evidence that neonatal outcomes are improved. Some aspects have not been evaluated in the trials reviewed, such as maternal satisfaction, infection rates and cost analysis, and further research is required before fetal blood sampling is recommended for practice.

Fetal electrocardiogram

Technology is available to monitor the fetal ECG during labour and studies have shown that the ST waveform is elevated in the presence of moderate to severe hypoxaemia (Greene 1987).There is some evidence to support the use of ST waveform analysis in conjunction with CEFM in labour (Neilson 2006; Amer-Walkin et al. 2007).

A review of the available literature by Neilson (2006) found that the incidence of operative deliveries, fetal blood sampling and severe metabolic acidosis at birth was reduced when ECG recordings were analysed in combination with interpretation of the CTG; however these data are from a very limited number of trials and should be treated with caution, as recommended by the author.

This technology does require the application of a scalp electrode to the fetal head, following rupture of the membranes, and is therefore invasive and may be unacceptable to some women in labour. The system may not detect pre-existing hypoxia (Pateman et al. 2008) and should not be used as an alternative to CEFM (Amer-Walkin et al. 2007). Neilson (2006) suggests initiating ST waveform analysis only if the CTG shows abnormal features. NICE recommends that a further randomised controlled trial should be undertaken (NCCWCH 2007).

Maternal and fetal electrocardiogram

Bhogal and Reinhard (2010) describe a new technology which allows the recording of the fetal and maternal ECG simultaneously via electrodes attached to the maternal abdomen. The CTG displays the fetal and maternal heart rate patterns in addition to the uterine activity and the authors discuss the possibility of eliminating confusion between maternal and fetal heart rate recording on the CTG during labour when there are signal deficiencies. Sherer et al. (2005) describe maternal heart rate changes with uterine contractions similar to fetal heart rate deceleration patterns.

This technique has not been evaluated and the efficacy and effectiveness are not known, although the authors recommend that consideration should be given to continual monitoring of the maternal pulse rate when CEFM is used (Bhogal and Reinhard 2010).

Fetal stimulation tests

There is little gold-standard evidence, i.e. from randomised controlled trials, regarding the use of fetal stimulation tests. Skupski et al. (2002) reported from a systematic review that there is observational evidence that digital stimulation of the fetal scalp can elicit reassuring fetal heart rate accelerations and is a good predictive test of fetal acidaemia. It is important to note that the absence of accelerations is not predictive of fetal acidosis. Incision of the fetal scalp during fetal blood sampling can also elicit a response, although this is only moderately predictive. NICE (NCCWCH 2007) recommends that digital stimulation of the fetal head during vaginal examination is a reasonable additional tool to CEFM for assessing fetal well-being in labour.

Fetal pulse oximetry

There is no evidence to suggest that the use of fetal pulse oximetry reduces overall caesarean section rates (East et al. 2007), although in one study there was a reduction in caesarean section when the CTG was non-reassuring (East et al. 2006).

The technique involves placing a sensor, attached by clip or suction, to the top of the fetal head or alongside the face or back during a vaginal examination. Again, this is an invasive procedure, but only one study (East et al. 2006) sought women's views and report limited discomfort with sensor placement and with the sensor in place during labour. Women did not report any additional movement restriction over and above that with CEFM in progress.

East et al. (2007) conclude that, on current evidence, a better method of evaluating fetal well-being in labour should be used and further research into fetal pulse oximetry is recommended. NICE (NCCWCH 2007) did not consider the technique in the publication of the *Intrapartum Care* guideline as it is not in current use in the UK.

CONCLUSION

Assessing fetal well-being in labour is complicated. The tools in use to aid detection of fetal compromise provide data which are at times difficult to interpret and subjective, with both inter- and intraobserver error, despite improved education. CEFM is associated with an increased rate of intervention during labour and operative delivery and should be restricted for use in high-risk cases (NCCWCH 2007), with IA recommended for low-risk women.

The aim of fetal heart rate monitoring remains the detection and appropriate management of fetal compromise to reduce the rates of long-term neurological damage. To this end clinical practice is informed by national guidelines (NCCWCH 2007) and, whilst new technologies are developed, care must be taken to ensure they are fully evaluated before being incorporated in to clinical care.

REFERENCES

Alfirevic, Z., Devane, D., & Gyte, G. M. (2006, September). Continuous cardiotocography (CTG) as a form of electronic fetal monitoring (EFM) for fetal assessment during labour. *Cochrane Database of Systematic Review* (3).

Allan, C., & Talbot, A. (2008). *Back to basics. Midwifery led training package for normality*. Birmingham: NHS West Midlands.

Altaf, S., Oppenheimer, C., & Shaw, R., et al. (2006). Practices and views on fetal heart monitoring: A structured observation and interview study. *British Journal of Obstetrics and Gynaecology, 113*, 409–418.

Amer-Walkin, I., Arulkumaran, S., & Hagberg, H., et al. (2007). Fetal electrocardiogram: ST waveform analysis in intrapartum surveillance. *British Journal of Obstetrics and Gynaecology, 114*, 1191–1193.

Armstrong, N. (2010). Clinical mentors' influence upon student midwives' clinical practice. *British Journal of Midwifery, 18*(2), 114–123.

Arulkumaran, S., & Chua, S. (1996). Cardiotocography in labour. *Current Obstetrics and Gynaecology*, 6(4), 182–188.

Ayres-de-Campos, D., Bernades, J., & Costa-Pereira, A., et al. (1999). Inconsistencies in classification by experts of cardiotocograms and subsequent clinical decisions. *British Journal of Obstetrics and Gynaecology, 106*, 1307–1310.

Association of Radical Midwives. (2000). Hearing variability. *Midwifery Matters.* (84) (Spring).

Beckley, S., Stenhouse, E., & Greene, K. (2000). The development and evaluation of a computer-assisted teaching programme for intrapartum fetal monitoring. *British Journal of Obstetrics and Gynaecology, 107*, 1138–1144.

Bhogal, K., & Reinhard, J. (2010). Maternal and fetal heart rate confusion during labour. *British Journal of Midwifery, 18*, 424–428.

Blake, D. (2008). Pinards: Out of use and out of date? *British Journal of Midwifery, 16*, 364–365.

Blincoe, A. J. (2005). Fetal monitoring challenges and choices for midwives. *British Journal of Midwifery, 13*, 108–111.

Blix, E., Sviggum, O., & Sofie Kass, K., et al. (2003). Inter-observer variation in assessment of 845 labour admission tests: Comparison between midwives and obstetricians in the clinical setting and two experts. *British Journal of Obstetrics and Gynaecology, 110*, 1–5.

Boos, A., Houghton-Jagger, M., & Paret, G. W., et al. (1995, December). A new lightweight fetal telemetry system. *Hewlett-Packard journal*, 82–93.

Confidential Enquiry into Maternal and Child Health. (2007). *Saving Mothers' Lives. Reviewing maternal deaths to make motherhood safer 2003–2005*. London: CEMACH.

Churchill, H., & Francome, C. (2009). British midwives' views on rising caesarean section rates. *British Journal of Midwifery, 17*, 774–778.

Confidential Enquiry into Stillbirths and Deaths in Infancy. (1997). *Fourth annual report*. London: Maternal and Child Health Research Consortium.

Department of Health. (2007). *Maternity matters: Choice, access and continuity of care in a safe service*. London: DOH.

Devane, D., & Lalor, J. (2005). Midwives' visual interpretation of intrapartum cardiotocographs: Intra and inter observer agreement. *Journal of Advanced Nursing, 52*, 133–141.

Devane, D., Smith, V., & Healy, P. (2010). Cardiotocography for assessment of fetal wellbeing during labour. *The Practising Midwife, 113*, 18–20.

Draycott, T., Winter, C., Crofts, J., & Barnfield, S. (Eds.). (2008). *PROMPT. Practical obstetric multi professional training course manual*. London: Royal College of Obstetricians and Gynaecologists.

East, C. E., Chan, F. Y., & Brenneck, E. S., et al. (2006). Women's evaluations of their experience in a multicenter randomized controlled trial of intrapartum fetal pulse oximetry (The Foremost Trial). *Birth, 33*, 101–109.

East, C. E., Chan, F. Y., & Colditz, P. B., et al. (2007). Fetal pulse oximetry for fetal assessment in labour. *Cochrane Database of Systematic Reviews* (2).

East, C. E., Leader, L. R., & Sheehan, P., et al. (2010). Intrapartum fetal scalp lactate sampling for fetal assessment in the presence of a non reassuring fetal heart rate trace. *Cochrane Database of Systematic Reviews* (3).

Eccles, M., Grimshaw, J., & Walker, A., et al. (2005). Changing the behavior of healthcare professionals: the use of theory in promoting the uptake of research findings. *Journal of Clinical Epidemiology, 58*, 105–112.

Ennis, M., & Vincent, C. A. (1990). Obstetric accidents: A review of 64 cases. *British Medical Journal, 300*, 1365–1367.

Fraser, J., & Blanas, K. (2007). The confident midwife. *The Practicing Midwife, 10*, 45–46.

Garcia, J., Corry, M., & MacDonald, D., et al. (1985). Mothers' views on continuous electronic fetal heart rate monitoring and intermittent auscultation in a randomised controlled trial. *Birth, 21*, 79–85.

GE Healthcare. (2010). Online. Available at: <www.gehealthcare.com/inen/monitor/products/telemetry/coro340-info.html> Accessed 10.07.10.

Greene, K. G. (1987). The ECG waveform. In M. Whittle (Ed.), *Baillière's clinical obstetrics and gynaecology* (Vol. 1, pp. 131–155). London: Baillière Tindall.

Hall, M. H. (2001). Caesarean section: *Why mothers die 1997–1999. The confidential enquiries into maternal deaths in the United Kingdom*. London: RCOG Press. pp. 317–325.

Harrison, J. (2004). Auscultation: The art of listening. *Midwives, 7*, 64–69.

Health Care Commission. (2007). *Women's experiences of maternity care in the NHS in England*. London: Health Care Commission.

Hindley, C., Wrenhinsliff, S. S., & Thompson, A. M. (2007). English midwives' views and experiences of intrapartum fetal heart rate monitoring in women at low obstetric risk: Conflicts and compromises. *Journal of Midwifery and Women's Health, 51*, 354–360.

Hollins Martin, C. J. (2008). Triumph over the barricades and put the evidence into practice. *British Journal of Midwifery, 16*, 76–81.

Ireland, J., Gibb, S., & West, B. C. (2008). Interprofessional education: Reviewing the evidence. *British Journal of Midwifery, 16*, 446–453.

MacDonald, D., Grant, A., & Sheridan-Pereira, M., et al. (1985). The Dublin randomised controlled trial of intrapartum fetal heart rate monitoring. *American Journal of Obstetrics and Gynecology, 52*, 524–539.

Mahomed, K., Nyoni, R., & Mulambo, T., et al. (1994). Randomised controlled trial of intrapartum fetal heart rate monitoring. *British Medical Journal, 308*, 497–500.

Mainstone, A. (2004). The use of doppler in fetal monitoring. *British Journal of Midwifery, 12*, 78–83.

McAra-Couper, J., Jones, M., & Smyth, E. (2010). Rising rates of intervention in childbirth. *British Journal of Midwifery, 18*, 160–169.

Medical Devices Agency. (2002). Cardiotocograph (CTG) monitoring of fetus during labour-update. Safety Notice MDS SN2002(23) August 2002. London: MDA.

Medicines and Healthcare products Regulatory Agency. (2010). Medical Device Alert ref MDA/2010/054. Online. Available at: <www.mhra.gov.uk/publications/safetywarning/medicaldevicealerts/CON085061> Accessed 10.07.10.

Mongelli, M., Chung, T. K. H., & Chang, A. M. Z. (1997). Obstetric intervention and benefit in conditions of very low prevalence. *British Journal of Obstetrics and Gynaecology, 104*, 771–774.

Munro, J., Ford, H., & Scott, A., et al. (2002). Action research project responding to midwives views of different methods of fetal monitoring in labour. *MIDIRS Midwifery Digest, 12*, 495–498.

National Colloborating Centre for Women's and Children's Health (NCCWCH). (2007). *Intrapartum Care. Care of healthy women and their babies during childbirth. Clinical Guideline*. London: RCOG Press.

National Institute for Health and Clinical Excellence. (2004). *Caesarean section, clinical guideline*. London: NICE.

Neilson, J. P. (2006). Fetal electrocardiogram (ECG) for fetal monitoring during labour. *Cochrane Database of Systematic Reviews* (3).

Neilson, D., Freeman, R., & Mangan, S. (2008). Signal ambiguity resulting in unexpected outcome with external fetal heart rate monitoring. *American Journal of Obstetrics and Gynacology, 198*, 717–724.

Nelson, K. B., Dambrosia, J. M., & Ting, T. Y., et al. (1996). Uncertain value of electronic fetal monitoring in predicting cerebral palsy. *New England Journal of Medicine, 334*, 613–618.

NHS Litigation Authority. (2009). *CNST Maternity clinical risk management standards*. London: DOH.

Nicholson, S., & Saunders, L. (2010). CNST maternity standards and assessments and other NHSLA risk management initiatives. *The Practising Midwife, 13*, 14–19.

Nursing and Midwifery Council. (2004). *Midwives rules and standards*. London: NMC.

Nursing and Midwifery Council. (2008). *The Code. Standards of conduct and performance and ethics for nurses and midwives*. London: NMC.

Pateman, K., Khalil, A., & O'Brien, P. (2008). Electronic fetal heart rate monitoring: Help or hindrance. *British Journal of Midwifery, 16*, 454–457.

Phillips Health Care. (2008). Online. Available at: <www.phillips.com/avalonCTS> Accessed 10.07.10.

Phillips Health Care. (2009). *Important device safety alert*. Online. Available at: <www.medical.phillips.com/us_en/support/fetal_monitor_notice.wpd> Accessed 07.07.01.

Royal College of Obstetricians and Gynaecologists. (2001a). *The national sentinel caesarean section audit report*. London: RCOG Press.

Royal College of Obstetricians and Gynaecologists. (2001b). *The use of electronic fetal monitoring. Evidence based guideline no 8*. London: RCOG Press.

Royal College of Obstetricians and Gynaecologists. (2007). *Safer Childbirth. Minimum standards for the organization and delivery of care in labour*. London: RCOG.

Saling, E., & Schneider, D. (1967). Biochemical supervision of the fetus during labour. *Journal of Obstetrics and Gynaecology of the British Commonwealth, 74*, 799–811.

Sherer, D., Dallou, L. M., & Pierre, N. (2005). Intrapartum repetitive maternal heart rate deceleration pattern simulating non reassuring fetal status. *American Journal of Perinatology, 22*, 165–167.

Skupski, D. W., Rosenberg, C. R., & Eglinton, G. S. (2002). Intrapartum fetal stimulation tests: a meta analysis. *Obstetrics and Gynaecology, 99*, 129–134.

Soltani, H., & Shallow, H. (2004). Re: Auscultation. *Letters Midwives, 7*, 172.

Supplee, R. B., & Vezeau, T. M. (1996). Continuous electronic fetal monitoring: does it belong in low-risk births? *American Journal of Maternal/Child Nursing, 21*, 301–306.

Thacker, S. B., Stroup, D. F., & Peterson, H. B. (1995). Efficacy and safety of intrapartum electronic fetal monitoring: An update. *Obstetrics and Gynaecology, 86*, 613–620.

Thacker, S. B., Stroup, D., & Chong, M. (2001). Continuous electronic heart rate monitoring for fetal assessment during labour. *The Cochrane Database of Systematic Reviews* (2).

Van Laar, J. O. E. H., Porath, M. M., & Peters, C. H. L., et al. (2008). Spectral analysis of fetal heart rate variability for fetal surveillance: review of the literature. *Acta Obstetrice et Gynecologica Scandanavica, 87*, 300–306.

Veerareddy, S., Khalil, A., & O'Brien, P. (2009). Obesity; Implications for labour and puerperium. *British Journal of Midwifery, 17*, 360–362.

Walsh, D. (2008). CTG use in intrapartum care; assessing the evidence. *Britsih Journal of Midwifery, 16*, 367–369.

Walsh, C. A., McMenamin, M. B., & Foley, M. E., et al. (2008). Trends in intrapartum fetal death 1979–2003. *American Journal of Obstetrics and Gynecology, 198*, 47–49.

Werkmeister, G. (2007). *Making normal birth a reality. Consensus statement from the maternity care working group.* London: National Childbirth Trust.

Interpretation of the CTG

PART 2

CONTROL OF THE FETAL HEART RATE

The mechanisms that control the fetal heart rate are complex and not completely understood. However it is important to have a basic understanding of what is known in order to appreciate why fetal heart rate abnormalities may be occurring and initiate appropriate management.

The heart beat originates in the sinoatrial node in the atrium and is controlled by the autonomic nervous system, primarily the sympathetic and parasympathetic pathways. Stimulation of the sympathetic pathway results in an increase in heart rate, whilst stimulation of the parasympathetic system, via the vagus nerve, will cause a decrease in the heart rate. The sympathetic system matures at a quicker rate than the parasympathetic, therefore exerting a stronger influence in the preterm fetus. Parasympathetic activity increases with gestational age and becomes dominant over other influences from 30 to 32 weeks' gestation, slowing the baseline heart rate (Serra et al. 2009).

The autonomic nervous system also responds to stimuli, via the midbrain, to baroreceptors and chemoreceptors.

Baroreceptors are found in the aorta and large arteries. They are sensitive to changes in arterial blood pressure. If the pressure increases parasympathetic activity is stimulated, resulting in a lowering of the heart rate.

Chemoreceptors are found in the midbrain and aorta and are sensitive to changes in the oxygen and carbon dioxide (CO_2) tension and hydrogen ion (H^+) concentration of the blood. A reduction in oxygen tension results in stimulation of the sympathetic pathway and an increase in heart rate.

Fetal oxygen supply

The fetus is reliant upon gaseous exchange at the placenta in order to maintain oxygen levels and eliminate CO_2. During labour gaseous exchange is affected by uterine contractions and umbilical cord compression. In order to adapt to these changes fetal blood has a high concentration of haemoglobin which in turn has a high affinity for oxygen. Fetal cardiac output is very efficient and under normal circumstances oxygen saturation is high and often exceeds requirements. Well-grown, term fetuses can compensate readily to temporary reductions in oxygen supply during labour.

The fetus uses oxygen to metabolise glucose and produce energy (aerobic metabolism). CO_2 is the waste product and is excreted via the placenta. During a contraction the CO_2 levels rise as a result of the impaired gaseous exchange and return to normal in between contractions. Prolonged impairment of gaseous exchange at the placenta will result in retention of CO_2. This will lead to the release of H^+ ions which are toxic to the fetus, and cause a fall in the pH of the blood (respiratory acidaemia). Fetal haemoglobin contains buffers which are able to mop up the H^+ ions, restoring the pH of the blood to normal levels. Bicarbonate ions (HCO_3^-) are also produced in the breakdown of CO_2 and act as another buffer which diffuses out of the blood vessels into the extracellular fluid.

In addition to an increase in CO_2 the oxygen tension of the blood will be decreased (hypoxaemia). If the oxygen levels fall to a critical level eventually supply to the tissues will be reduced (hypoxia). The fetus is able to rely on the following mechanisms in such circumstances:

- There is a greater extraction of oxygen from maternal blood at the placenta and the fetal tissues extract a greater proportion of oxygen from the fetal blood.
- Perfusion of the fetal heart, brain and adrenals is prioritised with a decrease in blood flow to the gut, kidneys and skin.
- The chemoreceptors detect a fall in the oxygen tension of the blood, activating a hormonal response. Levels of catecholamines released from the adrenal glands increase, resulting in a rise in the fetal heart rate and constriction of the peripheral blood vessels.
- Anaerobic (without oxygen) metabolism supplements energy supplies. This is achieved by the release of glucose from the fetal glycogen stores in the liver and muscle. It is broken down to form energy, with lactic acid as a byproduct. The buffers in the fetal haemoglobin and extracellular fluid will neutralise the lactic acid, although they do not have an infinite capacity and the pH of the fetal blood will continue to decrease (metabolic acidaemia).

Although the fetus is well equipped to compensate for a reduction in oxygen supply during labour, the resources required to maintain a normal pH of the blood are not inexhaustible. When they have been utilised or are in limited supply there is an increased risk of hypoxia and asphyxia (levels of oxygen low enough to cause damage to fetal tissue). A metabolic acidaemia cannot be corrected as readily as a respiratory acidaemia.

Fetal blood sampling

Testing of a sample of blood obtained from the fetal scalp can provide additional information when the cardiotocograph (CTG) has pathological features (NCCWHC 2007). It is possible to ascertain the pH value of the blood and also an estimate of the base deficit, the amount of available buffer that has been used up. This tends to be higher in metabolic acidaemia than respiratory acidaemia.

The decision to perform fetal blood sampling must be taken bearing in mind the clinical picture. In the event of acute fetal compromise delivery should be prepared for rather than delay the birth (NCCWHC 2007).

The results of the blood sample must also be interpreted after taking into account the progress being made in labour and the clinical condition of the woman and fetus.

pH	Interpretation of result
≥7.25	Normal
7.21–7.24	Borderline: repeat in 30 minutes or sooner if further CTG abnormalities
≤7.20	Abnormal: seek obstetric consultant advice. Prepare for delivery

Cord blood gas analysis

It is recommended (NCCWHC 2007) that paired cord blood samples are obtained when there has been a concern about the baby during labour or immediately after birth. However it is important to emphasise that the results are not a complete assessment of neonatal condition and must be interpreted alongside the condition of the baby, the Apgar scores and any resuscitation that has been necessary (K2 Medical Systems 2010). The results provide useful information for the exclusion of intrapartum-related hypoxic–ischaemic brain damage (NCCWHC 2007).

It is important that a paired sample of cord bloods is obtained from the umbilical artery and vein. The difference in pH between the arterial sample and venous sample can indicate the cause of the acidaemia. A large arteriovenous difference indicates an acute event or cord compression, whilst a small difference is more indicative of a chronic condition (K2 Medical Systems 2010).

An arterial pH of <7.05 and/or a venous pH <7.10 demonstrates evidence of acidaemia.

The base deficit distinguishes between a respiratory and metabolic acidaemia. An arterial base deficit of >12 mmol/l and/or a venous base deficit of >10 mmol/l is evidence of metabolic acidaemia.

Factors affecting oxygen supply and gaseous exchange

Any condition which affects the function of the placenta can in turn have an effect upon gaseous exchange and therefore the oxygen supply to the fetus. In pregnancies complicated by maternal hypertension, diabetes and pre-eclampsia, placental function can be compromised. The baby may be small for gestational age with reduced glycogen supplies and therefore an impaired capacity for compensating for a reduction in oxygen supply. Preterm babies are also at risk of compromise as they have not had the opportunity to lay down sufficient stores of glycogen. Placental abruption, uterine hypercontractility and uterine scar rupture will also reduce the level of gaseous exchange that is able to occur.

Any cord occlusion will prevent blood flow from the placenta to the fetus, such as cord prolapse, true knots or cords around limbs or neck of fetus. During a contraction the occlusion is intensified, resulting in a reduction or cessation of oxygen supply. Any condition of the fetus which involves a reduction in the oxygen-carrying capacity of the blood will increase the risk of hypoxia developing such as anaemia, twin-to-twin transfusion and infection, when oxygen requirements are raised.

INTERPRETATION OF THE CTG

Whilst the correct interpretation of the data on the CTG is important to assist with decisions regarding the management plan of labour it is vital that this information is not used in isolation (NCCWHC 2007). It is necessary to take into consideration any risk factors that have been identified both in the antepartum period and arising during the course of labour. For instance, it may be anticipated that a baby that is known to be small for gestational age at the onset of labour is more likely to have fetal heart rate abnormalities on the CTG once the added stress of uterine contractions begin than a well-grown baby. In addition, when labour requires augmentation with an oxytocic drug the fetus is at greater risk of developing abnormalities on the CTG as a result of the potential for hypercontractility.

The stage of labour, progress being made and strength and frequency of contractions, which must be recorded alongside the fetal heart rate, need to be assessed in addition to the presence and colour of liquor. Failure to observe all of these factors has been identified as a common error (Gibb 1997).

The terminology used to describe fetal heart rate patterns and the management of abnormalities must be consistent and in line with current national guidance (NCCWHC 2007; NHS Litigation Authority 2009a). All professionals who may be involved in CTG interpretation must be aware of these and attend regular training to maintain their knowledge and skills (NHS Litigation Authority 2009a). Barber et al. (2010) stress that CTG monitors are in fact recorders of data; the monitor is actually the healthcare professional who is interpreting that data and as such the quality of the interpretation is only as good as the ability of the professional to interpret it correctly. A recent study of stillbirth claims by the NHS Litigation Authority (2009b) demonstrated that misinterpretation of the CTG was the most frequent example of negligence found, with midwives being responsible in 70% of cases.

The CTG is a continual reflection of the fetal heart rate throughout labour. The data must be of good quality. A poor-quality CTG is of no use at all; fetal heart rate abnormalities may be missed or mistakenly identified, leading to inappropriate management. If difficulties are encountered monitoring the fetal heart with an abdominal transducer then application of a fetal scalp electrode should be considered following discussion with the woman.

As discussed previously, a number of factors can affect fetal oxygenation. It is therefore important that certain information is recorded upon the CTG contemporaneously.

- The CTG paper must be labelled with the name and identification number of the mother.
- The date and time of the recording must be documented. Most CTG monitors print out the date and time but this must be checked to ensure they are accurate, particularly at certain times of the year, when clocks move in and out of British summer time. In the event of a discrepancy the actual date and time must be written on the paper and the reason for the difference recorded alongside.
- The maternal pulse rate and auscultated fetal heart rate should be documented at the onset of the recording. This helps to confirm that it is the fetal heart rate that is being recorded.
- Any intrapartum events that may affect the fetal heart rate should be recorded, such as administration of drugs to the mother, including opiates and epidural analgesia, changes in maternal posture, vaginal examinations and their findings, rupture of the membranes and colour of liquor, application of a fetal scalp electrode, fetal blood sampling.
- If there is any concern about the rate of the fetal heart that is recording then the fetal heart rate should be auscultated with a Doppler or Pinard stethoscope and this rate documented on the CTG.

The CTG should be reviewed at least every hour during labour (NCCWHC 2007). The use of a pro forma such as that shown in Table 2.3 (see pp. 24) for classification and actions can aid practitioners to become familiar with and use standard terminology. If a practitioner is concerned about the interpretation of a CTG then a second opinion should be sought. Any midwife or doctor who provides an opinion on a CTG must sign the CTG and document his or her findings both on the CTG and in the case notes, noting the date and time. The CTG should be categorised as normal, suspicious or pathological. A plan of care should always be made for further management and when the CTG should be reviewed again and by whom. Discussions must always take place with the woman and her partner to explain to them the reasons for any concerns, why they may be occurring and what plan will be put into place, including the risks and benefits of any additional tests such as fetal blood sampling that may be suggested.

CTGs must be stored safely within the woman's case notes following birth.

FEATURES OF THE CARDIOTOCOGRAPH

In order to interpret a CTG, there are four main features to consider relating to the fetal heart rate:

Basic patterns

1. baseline heart rate
2. variability.

Periodic changes

3. accelerations
4. decelerations.

In normal circumstances:

- The baseline fetal heart rate is 110–160 bpm.
- The variability is 5–15 beats.
- Accelerations may or may not occur in response to uterine contractions or fetal movements.
- No decelerations occur.

Figure 2.1 shows an example of a normal CTG.

BASIC PATTERNS

Baseline fetal heart rate

This is estimated over a 5–10-minute period of CTG excluding accelerations or decelerations and is recorded in beats per minute (bpm). In normal circumstances the baseline fetal heart rate is 110–160 bpm. It is important to note the baseline rate at the beginning of the CTG; a gradual rise in baseline, although still remaining within the normal range, is suspicious (NCCWHC 2007).

Baseline bradycardia

Definition

Baseline bradycardia is defined as being a persistently low baseline of below 110 bpm.

Causes

Many baseline bradycardias have no identifiable cause but certain factors need to be taken into consideration:

- Gestational age of greater than 40 weeks. Some postmature fetuses have a marked vagal tone, causing a slowing of the heart rate, and can show a baseline bradycardia of 100–110 bpm.
- Cord compression. In cases of acute hypoxia and cord compression a change in heart rate can be evident from within a normal range to a bradycardia that does not recover to the baseline.
- Congenital heart malformations.
- Certain drugs, e.g. benzodiazepines.

Baseline tachycardia

Definition

Baseline tachycardia is defined as being a persistently high baseline of above 160 bpm. A baseline heart rate

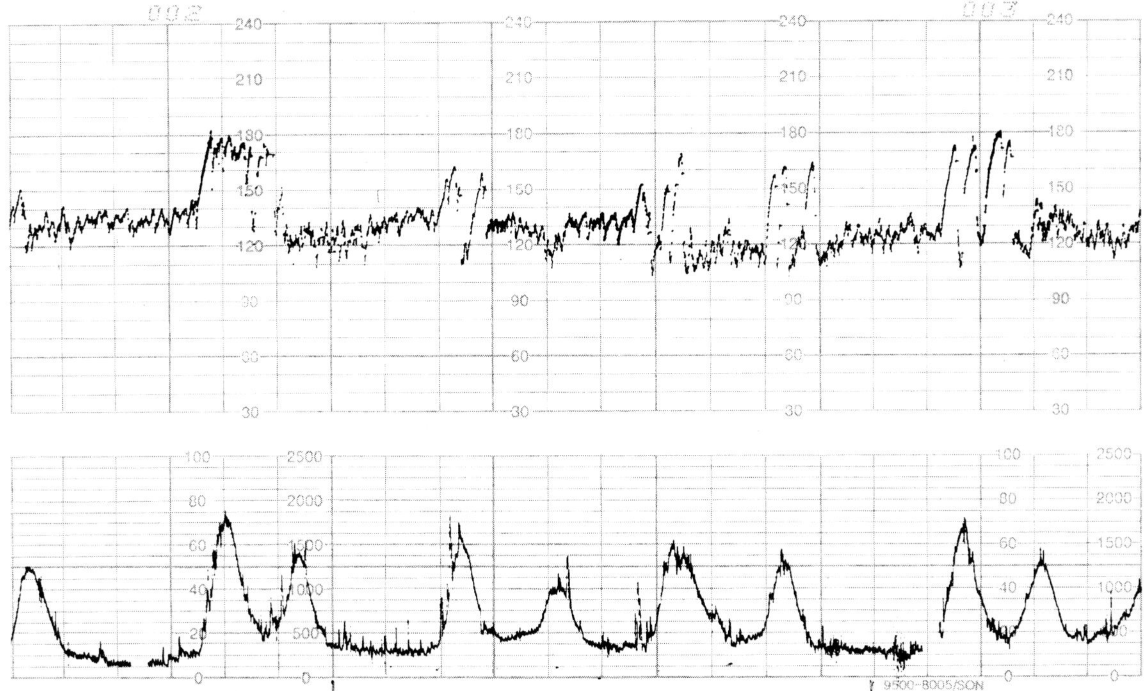

Fig. 2.1 *Normal CTG. Fetal heart recorded using fetal scalp electrode. Contractions recorded using an external transducer. Baseline 125–135 bpm; baseline variability 5–15 bpm; no decelerations; accelerations with some contractions.*

of 160–180 bpm where accelerations are present and no adverse features are identified should be regarded as normal, an uncomplicated baseline tachycardia (NCCWHC 2007).

Causes

1. Excessive fetal movements or fetal stimulation. If the fetus is very active during the period when the CTG is being performed, the fetal heart may not be showing a true baseline. This should be classed as reactivity, but can be mistakenly diagnosed as fetal tachycardia.
2. Maternal stress and anxiety. If the mother is in a stressful situation, or has a high anxiety level, she will release catecholamines, thereby stimulating the sympathetic nervous system, resulting in an increase in both maternal and fetal heart rates.
3. Gestational age. A fetus at a gestational age of 32 weeks or below can show a baseline tachycardia due to the immaturity of the vagus nerve. The sympathetic nervous system is dominant, resulting in a persistently high fetal heart rate (Ingemarsson et al. 1993).
4. Maternal tachycardia. This may be as a result of dehydration and/or ketosis leading to poor uterine perfusion. Encouraging fluids, isotonic drinks and appropriate diet would be recommended.
5. Maternal pyrexia. A maternal pyrexia of 37.5 °C or higher may indicate infection and possible chorioamnionitis and is a risk factor for poor neonatal outcome (Impey et al. 2008).
6. Fetal infection. During infection, oxygen requirements are raised. The heart rate rises to increase the oxygen transfer around the body.
7. Fetal hypoxia. Chronic changes in the levels of oxygen tension in the blood and fetal tissues lead to an increase in the sympathetic activity, resulting in a rise in heart rate.
8. Fetal hormones. The fetus, in response to stressful situations, e.g. a decrease in oxygen levels, can produce hormones from the adrenal glands, adrenaline (epinephrine) and noradrenaline (norepinephrine). Their effect is similar to an increase in sympathetic activity, that is, a rise in the heart rate.

Management

Record maternal temperature and pulse rate. If pyrexial then tepid sponging and administration of paracetamol and antibiotics may be considered. In the absence of any other fetal heart rate abnormalities the CTG should be observed and reviewed regularly in line with labour progress.

If other fetal heart rate abnormalities are present, suggesting fetal compromise, then fetal blood sampling may be performed providing there are no contraindications to the procedure.

Variability

Definition

Variability is due to interaction between all the systems previously described and occurs as a result of the beat-to-beat changes in the heart rate. Normal variability is 5–15 bpm (Fig. 2.1). Variability <5 bpm is classed as reduced.

Variability can be measured by analysing a 1-minute portion of a CTG, and assessing the amplitude of change in the heart rate during that period, i.e. the difference in the number of beats per minute of the fetal heart from the highest rate to the lowest rate (any accelerations and decelerations should be excluded, e.g. if the highest rate is 160 bpm and the lowest rate is 155 bpm the difference is 5 bpm).

Aetiology

Variability represents the constant interaction of the sympathetic and parasympathetic nervous systems as they determine the appropriate heart rate and cardiac output in response to constant minor changes in venous return and metabolic demands of the fetus (Samueloff et al. 1994). Normal variability represents an intact nervous pathway through the cerebral cortex, midbrain, vagus nerve and cardiac conduction system. Variability is likely to occur as a result of numerous inputs transmitted through these areas of the nervous system.

Decreased variability

Causes

1. Fetal sleep. During fetal sleep the CTG commonly gives an appearance of decreased variability; this should not be confused with lack of reactivity. The pattern does not usually persist for longer than 40 minutes, although it may last for up to 90 minutes (Spencer and Johnson 1986).
2. Administration of drugs to the mother. Decreased variability can be seen following the administration of pethidine for pain relief in labour, or of sedative drugs. This pattern may persist for longer than the normal sleep cycle of the fetus (Gibb and Arulkumaran 2008).
3. Gestational age. The CTG of a fetus at a gestational age of less than 30–32 weeks may show decreased variability, probably due to the immaturity of the autonomic nervous system (Serra et al. 2009).
4. Hypoxia. When the fetus is suffering from hypoxia the autonomic nervous system fails to respond to stress and the changes in venous return and metabolic demands of the fetus. This is due to a reduction in the transmission of impulses through the nervous system. In the presence of cerebral hypoxia, variability is often severely diminished or absent (McMurtry Baird and Ruth 2002).

Management

When diminished variability is diagnosed on a CTG, providing any obvious causes, such as administration of pethidine, can be eliminated, fetal hypoxia must always be considered as a cause. Fetal blood sampling should be performed to assess the pH value and base excess of the blood.

Sinusoidal pattern

Definition

These patterns are identifiable by the smooth, undulating, sine wave-like baseline. Variability is absent. The amplitude of the undulations is usually 5–15 beats and the frequency 2–5 per minute (McMurty Baird and Ruth 2002). O'Connor et al. (1980), following a review of the literature, note that sinusoidal tracings, where the oscillations have an amplitude of 20 beats or more, and a frequency of 1–2 oscillations per minute, are more suggestive of fetal hypoxia and are an indication for immediate delivery.

Sinusoidal traces, where the amplitude of the oscillations is 10 beats or less, with a frequency of 3–5 per minute, may be due to fetal anaemia or thumb-sucking. They can be referred to as pseudosinusoidal and do not usually require immediate action. However, if other fetal heart rate abnormalities are present, delivery should not be delayed.

Sinusoidal patterns are uncommon and a true sinusoidal pattern is associated with a poor neonatal outcome (Schneider and Tropper 1986). Figure 2.2 shows an example CTG exhibiting a sinusoidal pattern.

Aetiology

It is thought that this pattern may be a result of cord compression, resulting in alternating hypervolaemia and hypovolaemia, or of a raised intraperitoneal pressure due to the presence of ascites, resulting in a reduction and eventual cessation of umbilical venous blood flow. In both instances, significant fetal hypoxia will result (O'Connor et al. 1980).

A fetus with anaemia, as a result of rhesus incompatibility, twin-to-twin transfusion or a large fetal bleed such as ruptured vasa praevia, may produce a sinusoidal pattern, reflecting hypoxia.

This pattern can also be seen as a result of fetal thumb-sucking, and is sometimes seen following the administration of narcotic analgesia, particularly pethidine, to the mother (Egley et al. 1991). In these cases the variability will have been normal initially and

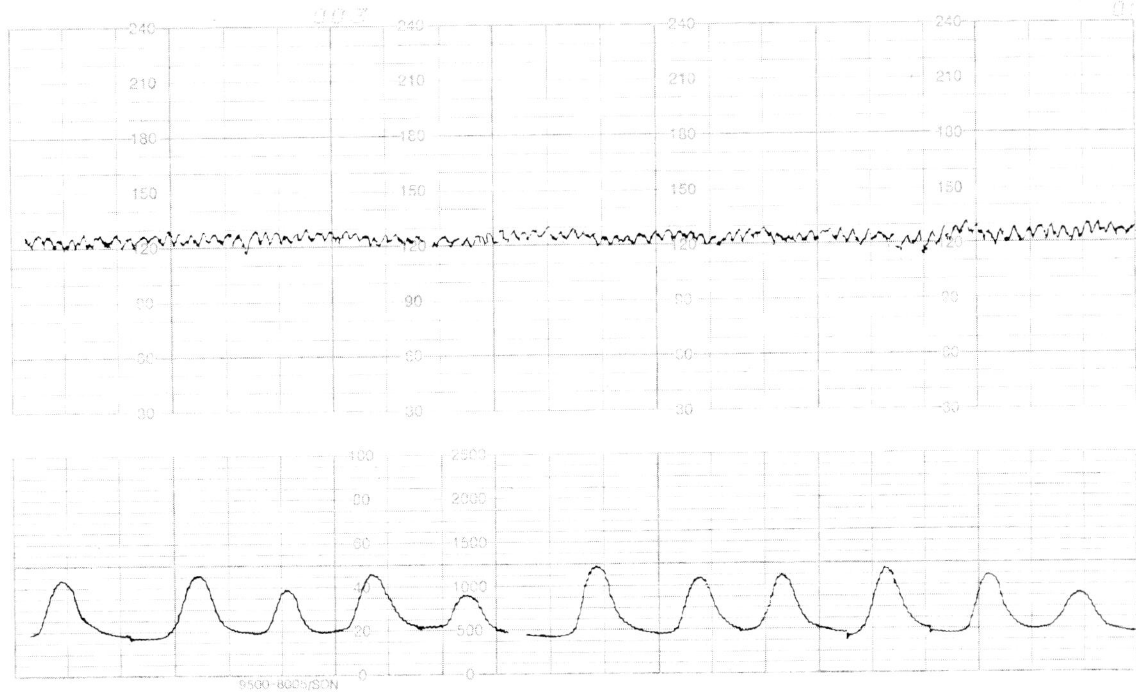

Fig. 2.2 *Sinusoidal pattern.*

the pattern should not persist for longer than 40 minutes before there is a return to normal variability. If the pattern persists then fetal blood sampling should be performed.

PERIODIC CHANGES

Accelerations

Definition

An acceleration is an increase in the fetal heart rate of 15 bpm or more, lasting for at least 15 seconds. Accelerations usually occur in response to either a fetal movement or a uterine contraction. When accelerations occur the CTG is said to be reactive and they are a reassuring sign, even in the presence of decreased variability (NCCWHC 2007). When accelerations are absent on an otherwise reassuring CTG the significance is uncertain (Draycott et al. 2008); however absence of accelerations along with a decrease in variability and/or an increase in heart rate is more suggestive of a hypoxic response (Gibb and Arulkumaran 2008).

Aetiology

The reaction is caused by the interaction of the sympathetic and parasympathetic nervous systems as a result of an increase in metabolic demands of the fetus during an active phase, or during a uterine contraction in response to compression of the umbilical cord and fetal trunk.

Increased reactivity

This can be due to a period of excessive fetal movements. On analysis of the CTG, increased reactivity can be mistakenly identified as baseline tachycardia.

Decreased reactivity

This can be due to either a period of fetal sleep or the administration of sedation or analgesia to the mother. Methods of fetal stimulation, such as abdominal palpation or giving the mother cold water to drink, can evoke a response in the fetus.

It is important not to confuse decreased reactivity with decreased variability. A CTG can be non-reactive but still show variability within normal limits.

Decelerations

Decelerations of the fetal heart rate from the baseline can be classified into four types:

1. early
2. late
3. variable
4. prolonged.

The definition and physiological explanation for each type of deceleration are different. It is important to classify them accurately in order for the most effective management to be initiated. Uterine contractions must be monitored adequately in order for the deceleration to be classified.

Early decelerations

Definition

Early decelerations tend to be uniform in shape and occur with each contraction. They often appear in a mirror image of the contraction. The onset of the deceleration is at the onset of the contraction. The heart rate reaches its lowest point at the peak of the contraction and has recovered to the baseline by the end of the contraction. The amplitude of the deceleration is usually 40 bpm or less. True early decelerations are rare and are not associated with hypoxia (NCCWHC 2007).

Figure 2.3 shows an example CTG exhibiting early decelerations.

Aetiology

Early decelerations are caused by compression of the fetal head during a contraction. They are seen in late first stage of labour. Compression of the fetal head causes an increase in intracranial pressure and therefore a decrease in cerebral blood flow and oxygenation. The decrease in oxygen tension is detected by cerebral chemoreceptors, and parasympathetic activity is increased, resulting in a fall in the fetal heart rate. During head compression, pressure on the vagal centre in the brain may also occur, increasing parasympathetic activity. A change in maternal posture will often relieve the pressure. Because early decelerations are rare, if they are identified on a CTG it is worth having a second thought. They are often confused with variable decelerations and the physiology, effect on the fetus and management are very different.

Late decelerations

Definition

Late decelerations are usually uniform in shape and depth and occur after each contraction. Any deceleration whose lowest point occurs more than 15 seconds after the peak of the contraction is said to be late (for an example CTG, see Fig. 2.4).

Aetiology

Late decelerations arise as a result of a decrease in uterine blood flow and therefore oxygen transfer during a uterine contraction. The low oxygen tension is detected by chemoreceptors in the aortic arch, resulting in stimulation of the parasympathetic pathways and an increase in vagal activity, leading to a fall in the

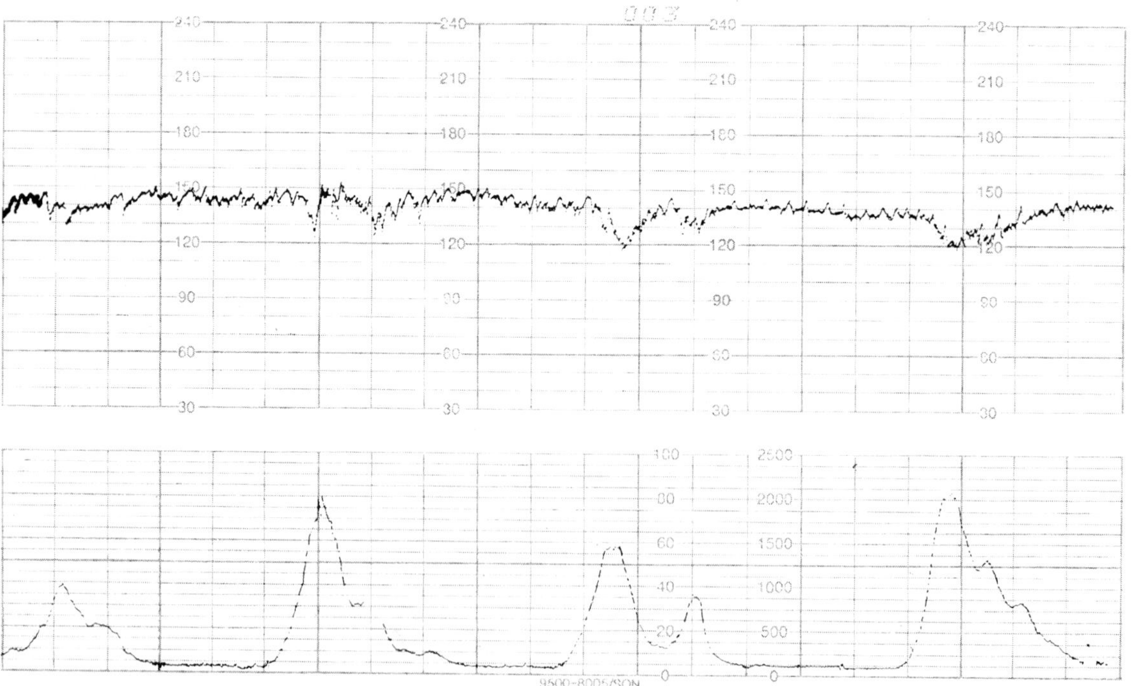

Fig. 2.3 *Early decelerations.*

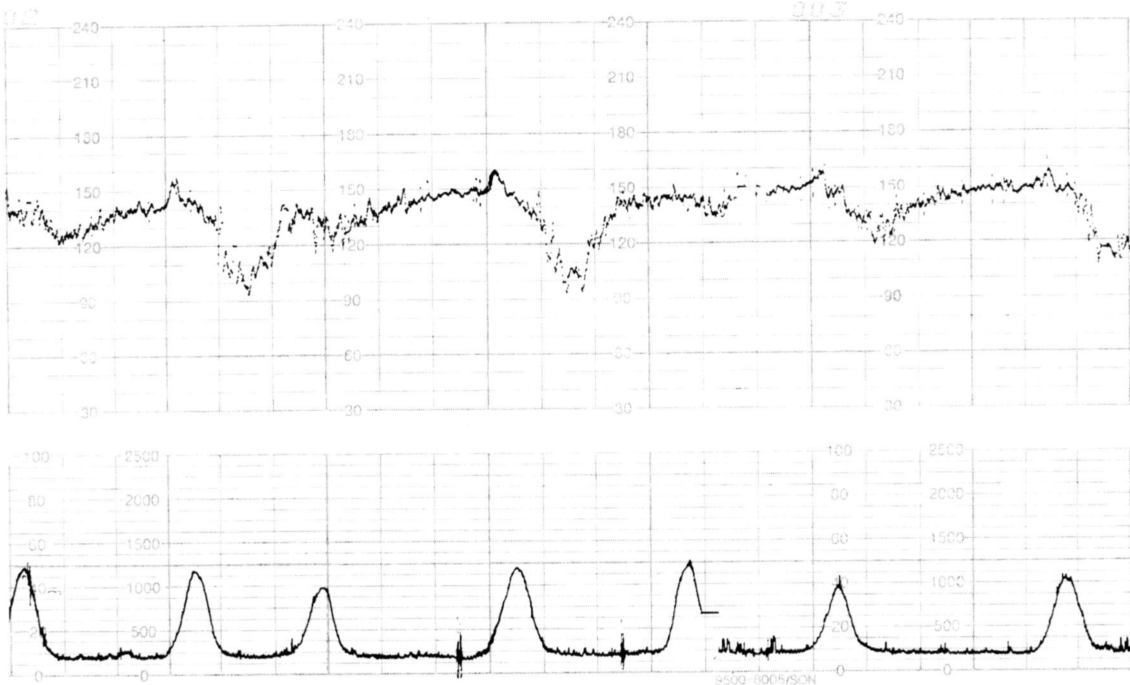

Fig. 2.4 *Late decelerations.*

heart rate. The decelerations occur after the contraction owing to the time it takes for the circulating blood to reach the aortic arch from the placenta. In between the contractions the rate of oxygen transfer between the placenta and the fetus is adequate, and the fetal heart rate baseline and variability are normal, indicating adequate cerebral oxygenation. If, however, the fetus is already compromised, then the reduced amount of oxygen transferred during a contraction may not be sufficient to maintain myocardial activity. Direct myocardial depression occurs, in addition to an increase in vagal activity. The rate of oxygen transfer in between the contractions may not be sufficient to maintain adequate oxygenation, which will be characterised by a decrease, or absence, of variability and, eventually, baseline tachycardia. Late decelerations that persist for 30 minutes or longer are indicative of hypoxia.

Causes

Any condition which causes a reduction in placental blood flow may result in late decelerations, for example:

- placental abruption
- maternal hypotension
- excessive uterine activity.

In addition, any maternal or pregnancy-related disease which may result in placental pathology can also cause late decelerations, for example:

- diabetes mellitus
- pregnancy-induced hypertension.

Any fetus that is already compromised, by either lack of stored glycogen or a reduction in circulating red blood cells for the transfer of oxygen, is also at an increased risk of developing late decelerations:

- intrauterine growth retardation
- prematurity
- rhesus isoimmunisation
- twin-to-twin transfusion.

Management

The aim is to increase the uterine blood flow and oxygen transfer across the placenta to the fetus.

1. Change maternal posture, preferably to left lateral.
2. Increase or commence intravenous infusion.
3. Stop any oxytocic infusion, if in progress to correct uterine hypercontractility. Administration of a tocolytic drug such as terbutaline may be considered if an oxytocin infusion is not in use (NCCWHC 2007).
4. A fetal blood sample should be obtained to assess the pH value and base excess of the fetal blood.
5. Whilst the above actions are being undertaken, the mother should be prepared for delivery, particularly if the baseline variability is decreased or if baseline

tachycardia or bradycardia develops in between the decelerations.

Variable decelerations

Definition

Variable decelerations are inconsistent in shape and frequency and in their relationship to uterine contractions. They are common and most decelerations that occur in labour are variable (NCCWHC 2007). They tend to have an amplitude of 40 bpm or more. Typical variable decelerations have shoulders – accelerations on either side of the deceleration. This demonstrates a normal physiological response to cord compression and is a reassuring feature (Gibb and Arulkumaran 2008).

Figure 2.5 shows an example CTG exhibiting variable decelerations.

Atypical variable decelerations are more indicative of fetal compromise developing (Fig. 2.6). They can be characterised by a number of features:

- loss of shouldering
- delayed recovery of fetal heart to baseline following deceleration
- rebound tachycardia
- reduction in variability during deceleration
- biphasic deceleration
- tend to be of greater depth and longer-lasting

Aetiology

Variable decelerations appear to occur as the result of transient compression of the umbilical cord, between the fetus and surrounding maternal tissues or fetal parts, during a uterine contraction.

During a uterine contraction, venous return is obstructed, leading to a decrease in venous return to the fetal heart. This in turn results in a decrease in cardiac output, and therefore arterial pressure. The baroreceptors in the aortic arch are stimulated and sympathetic activity is increased, resulting in a rise in the fetal heart rate to maintain the blood pressure. With further cord compression, the arterial flow becomes obstructed and fetal hypertension results. The baroreceptors in the aortic arch are stimulated, this time resulting in increased parasympathetic activity, leading to a fall in the fetal heart rate, also in an attempt to maintain the blood pressure at a normal level. The deceleration now occurs. As the contraction subsides and the arterial flow obstruction is removed, fetal hypotension recurs until the venous flow returns to normal. A reactionary tachycardia develops. When the contraction has ended, venous flow returns to normal and the fetal heart rate returns to the baseline.

The effect of variable decelerations upon the fetus varies depending upon the duration and degree of cord occlusion that occurs during a contraction. The longer the deceleration lasts, and the greater the amplitude, the more suggestive it is of fetal compromise. However, the baseline

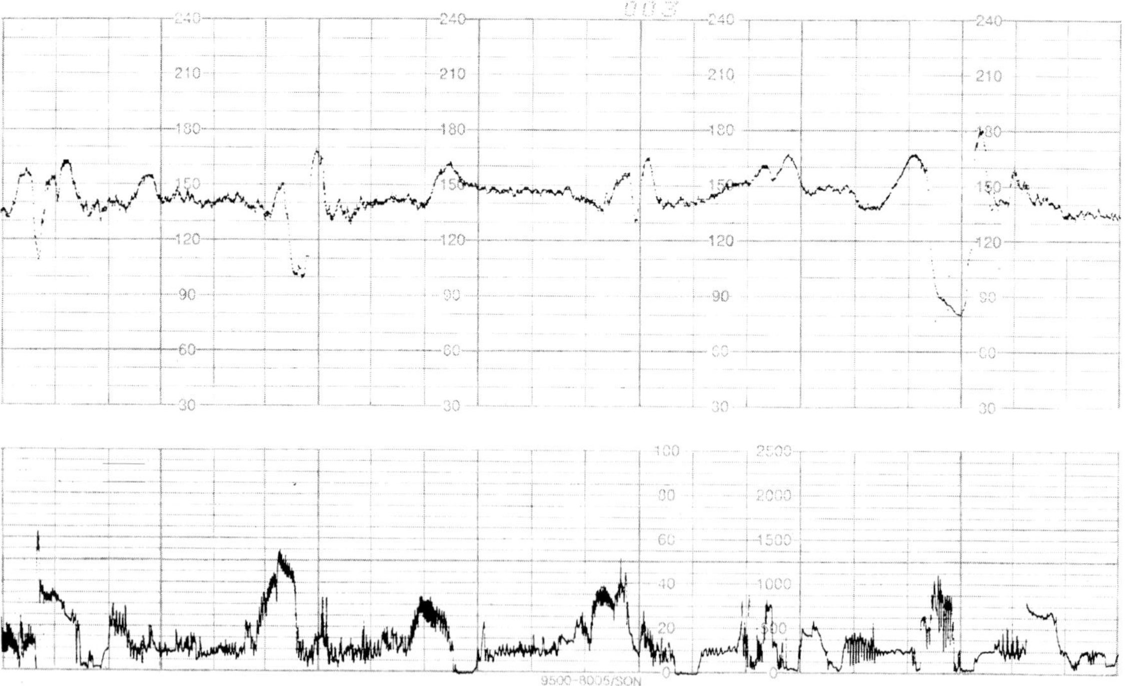

Fig. 2.5 *Variable decelerations.*

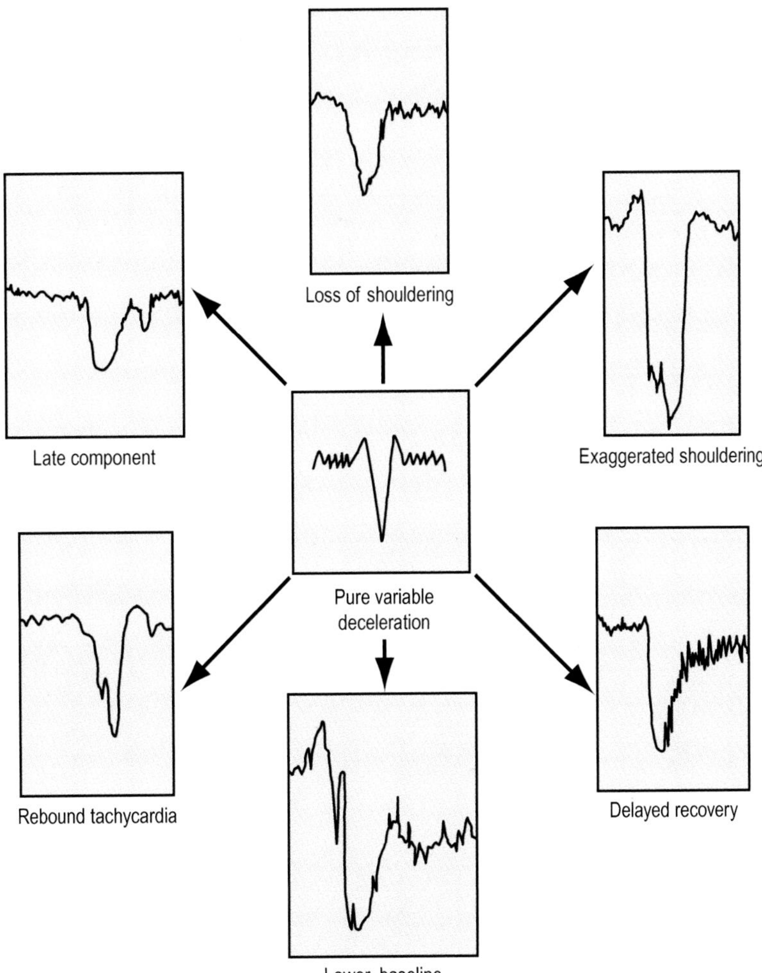

Fig. 2.6 *Diagrammatic representation of atypical variable decelerations.* Reproduced with permission from; Draycott T, Winter C, Crofts J et al. PROMPT: Practical Obstetric Multiprofessional Training Course Manual. London: RCOG Press, 2008. Copyright PROMPT Foundation.

of the fetal heart and the variability in between the decelerations are the best indicators of fetal oxygenation.

Causes

Variable decelerations are commonly seen when there is any form of umbilical cord entanglement, for example:

- umbilical cord around the neck or body
- true knot in the umbilical cord
- prolapsed umbilical cord.

Management

This is aimed at attempting to relieve the cord compression:

1. Change the maternal position, preferably to left lateral.
2. Carry out a vaginal examination to exclude cord prolapse if this is deemed to be a possibility.
3. Stop any oxytocic infusion, if in progress.
4. Increase intravenous fluids.
5. If the decelerations are atypical, the variability in between them is reduced or baseline tachycardia or bradycardia develops, fetal blood sampling should be performed to assess the pH value and base excess of the blood. The mother should be prepared for delivery while this is being performed.

Prolonged deceleration

Definition

A prolonged deceleration is described as consisting of a drop in the fetal heart rate of 30 bpm or more, lasting for a period of at least 2 minutes (for an example CTG, see Fig. 2.7). If the deceleration persists for 3 minutes or longer then plans should be made to expedite the delivery (NCCWHC 2007).

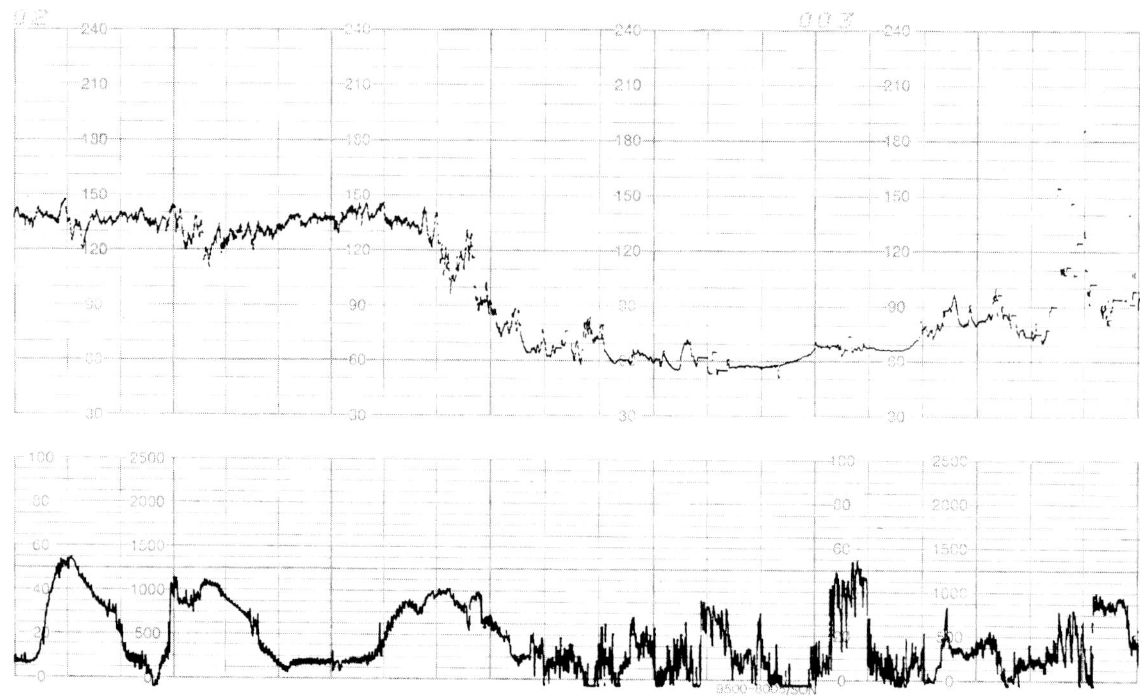

Fig. 2.7 *Prolonged deceleration.*

Aetiology

Prolonged decelerations are caused by a decrease in oxygen transfer across the placenta to the fetus, usually as a result of a decrease in uterine blood flow. The chemoreceptors in the aortic arch are stimulated, resulting in an increase in parasympathetic activity and a fall in fetal heart rate.

Causes

1. Total umbilical cord occlusion, e.g. cord prolapse.
2. Maternal hypotension resulting from the administration of local anaesthetic via an epidural catheter.
3. Uterine hypercontractility.
4. Prolonged decelerations can also be evident following vaginal examination or artificial rupture of the membranes. This could be due to direct pressure being applied on to the fetal head, resulting in pressure on the vagal centre in the brain.

Management

This is aimed at increasing blood flow to the uterus, and oxygen transfer across the placenta to the fetus, in addition to ascertaining the cause of the deceleration:

1. Change the maternal position to left lateral in the first instance.
2. Increase intravenous fluids.
3. Stop oxytocic infusion, if in progress.
4. Carry out a vaginal examination to exclude cord prolapse.
5. Assess maternal blood pressure, particularly if an epidural block is in progress.
6. Prepare the mother for delivery while the above actions are being performed.
7. Obtain a fetal blood sample on recovery of the fetal heart rate to the baseline to assess the pH value and base excess of the blood. If this is performed during the deceleration, then a transient acidosis will be present, but may not be a true reflection of the degree of fetal hypoxia.

If the CTG has been normal beforehand, a definite cause can be attributed to the deceleration, appropriate management is initiated and the fetal heart rate returns to normal, the fetal outcome is usually good. If the variability is decreased, or any other fetal heart rate abnormalities are present, then this is more suggestive of significant fetal hypoxia.

INTERPRETATION OF THE DATA

As noted previously, standardisation of terminology is important when interpreting a CTG. Current guidance recommends that fetal heart rate features are categorised using the templates shown in Tables 2.1 and 2.2.

All professionals who interpret the CTG and record their observations in the case notes and on the CTG paper must use consistent and correct terminology. Table 2.3 illustrates an example of a pro forma for the classification of a CTG and subsequent action. Routine use of such a tool encourages midwives, doctors and students to become familiar with terminology and appropriate management of fetal heart rate abnormalities. The interpretation of the CTGs in Part 4 is aided by the use of this pro forma.

MANAGEMENT OF A SUSPICIOUS CTG

A CTG categorised as suspicious will have one of the features in the non-reassuring section. Management will be conservative and should include:

- Maternal observations. Is there a pyrexia that requires treatment or a tachycardia that may be due to dehydration? Is the blood pressure normal?
- Maternal position. Is she lying supine? If so, suggest adopting a left lateral position.
- Has there been any recent intervention, such as a vaginal examination or rupture of the membranes? Has the woman been vomiting or suffered a vasovagal episode?

Obstetric and delivery shift leader review should be requested and a management plan agreed following discussion with the woman and her partner. This must be documented in the case notes. The CTG should be observed for any further abnormalities.

Table 2.1 Definition of normal, suspicious and pathological fetal heart rate traces

Category	Definition
Normal	All four features are classified as reassuring
Suspicious	One feature is classified as non-reassuring and the remaining features are classified as reassuring
Pathological	Two or more features are classified as non-reassuring or one or more classified as abnormal

MANAGEMENT OF A PATHOLOGICAL CTG

A pathological CTG will have either two or more features in the non-reassuring category or one or more in the abnormal section. The aim now is either to exclude hypoxia by fetal blood sampling or to expedite delivery if fetal blood sampling is inappropriate. This may be due to the inability to obtain a sample of blood if the cervical os is not dilated sufficiently or as a result of poor technique or if the fetal heart rate abnormality is deemed too severe to delay birth.

During the time that preparations for birth are being made the woman should be encouraged to adopt the left lateral position and intravenous fluids should be given if the blood pressure is low.

The debate surrounding the administration of facial oxygen to the woman when there are non-reassuring features on a CTG continues. A systematic review in 2003 concluded that there was insufficient evidence to support

Table 2.2 Classification of fetal heart rate trace features

Feature	Baseline (bpm)	Variability (bpm)	Decelerations	Accelerations
Reassuring	110–160	≥5	None	Present
Non-reassuring	100–109 161–180	<5 for 40–90 minutes	Typical variable decelerations with over 50% of contractions, for over 90 minutes Single prolonged deceleration for up to 3 minutes	The absence of accelerations with otherwise normal trace is of uncertain significance
Abnormal	<100 >180 Sinusoidal pattern ≥10 minutes	<5 for 90 minutes	Either atypical variable decelerations with over 50% of contractions or late decelerations, both for over 30 minutes Single prolonged deceleration for more than 3 minutes	

Reproduced with permission from National Institute for Health and Clinical Excellence (NICE) (2007) CG55. Intrapartum care: care of healthy women and their babies during childbirth. London: NICE. Available at: www.nice.org.uk/guidance/CG55.

Table 2.3 Pro forma for the classification of a cardiotocograph (CTG) and subsequent action

North Bristol NHS trust	Reassuring	Non-reassuring	Abnormal	Comments
Baseline rate	110–160 bpm	100–109 bpm 161–180 bpm	Less than 100 bpm Over 180 bpm Sinusoidal pattern for 10 minutes or more	
Variability	5 bpm or more	Less than 5 bpm for 40–90 minutes (in the absence of accelerations)	Less than 5 bpm for 90 minutes (in the absence of accelerations)	
Accelerations	Present	Comments:		
Decelerations	None	Typical variable decelerations with over 50% of contractions for over 90 minutes Single prolonged deceleration up to 3 minutes	Atypical variable decelerations with over 50% of contractions for over 30 minutes Late decelerations for over 30 minutes Single prolonged deceleration more than 3 minutes	
Opinion	Normal CTG (all four features reassuring)	Suspicious CTG (one non-reassuring feature)	Pathological CTG (two or more non-reassuring or one or more abnormal features)	
Dilatation (cm)	Cont's :10	Liquor colour	Mat pulse	
Action				
Date .... Time....................	Signature..		Status..	

Reproduced with permission from: Draycott T, Winter C, Crofts J et al. PROMPT: Practical Obstetric Multiprofessional Training Course Manual. London: RCOG Press, 2008. Copyright PROMPT Foundation.

this treatment (Fawole and Hofmeyr 2003). A more recent study, although acknowledged as small, reported findings which supported the use of oxygen (Haydon et al. 2006). The National Institute for Health and Clinical Excellence concludes that there is no evidence available that evaluates the risks and benefits with the short-term use of facial oxygen in the management of fetal heart rate abnormalities (NCCWHC 2007) and it is not currently recommended in clinical practice for the management of fetal heart rate abnormalities.

It is important that all practitioners are familiar with recent evidence relating to fetal monitoring in labour and that recommendations are incorporated into clinical guidelines within individual trusts. Regular training and updating must be accessible for all midwives, doctors and students and attendance monitored. CTG interpretation is subjective, although the introduction and routine use of a pro forma as in Table 2.3 should assist with consistency of interpretation and actions. Some trusts have implemented a system whereby a different midwife/doctor reviews the CTG at hourly intervals, whilst others routinely have two practitioners to review the CTG together. The emphasis remains the safety of women and babies and the detection and initiation of appropriate management of fetal heart rate abnormalities to reduce the perinatal mortality and morbidity rates related to intrapartum hypoxia.

REFERENCES

Barber, V. S., Lean, K. A., & Shakeshaft, C. E. (2010). Computers and CTGs: Where are we at? *British Journal of Midwifery, 18*, 644–649.

Draycott, T., Winter, C., & Crofts, J. et. al. (Eds.), (2008). *PROMPT. Practical Obstetric Multi Professional Training Course Manual*. London: RCOG.

Egley, C C, Bowes, W A, Jr, & Wagner, D (1991). Sinusoidal fetal heart rate pattern during labor. *American Journal of Perinatology, 8*, 197–220.

Fawole, B, & Hofmeyr, G. J. (2003). Maternal oxygen administration for fetal distress (Cochrane review): *The Cochrane library*. Oxford Update software.

Gibb, D (1997). Really understanding the cardiotocograph (CTG). *Professional Care of Mother and Child, 7*, 125–128.

Gibb, D, & Arulkumaran, S. (2008). *Fetal monitoring in practice* (3rd ed.). Edinburgh: Elsevier.

Haydon, M. L., Gorenberg, D. M., & Nageotte, M. P., et al. (2006). The effect of maternal oxygen administration on fetal pulse oximetry during labor in fetuses with non-reassuring fetal heart rate patterns. *American Journal of Obstetrics and Gynecology, 195*, 75–79.

Impey, L. W. M., Greenwood, C. E. L., & Black, P. S., et al. (2008). The relationship between intrapartum maternal fever and neonatal acidosis as risk factors for neonatal encephalopathy. *American Journal of Obstetrics and Gynecology, 198*, 49–51.

Ingemarsson, I., Ingemarsson, E., & Spencer, J. A. D. (1993). *Fetal heart rate monitoring. A practical guide*. Oxford: Oxford Medical Publications.

K2 Medical Systems. (2010). *Fetal Monitoring Training Package*. Online. Available at: <http://training.K2ms.com/content_VO13/locale_3/CBGChapter/start.htm/> Accessed 04.07.10.

McMurty Baird, S., & Ruth, D. J. (2002). Electronic fetal monitoring of the preterm fetus. *Journal of Perinatology and Neonatal Nursing, 16*, 12–24.

National Collborating Centre for Women's and Children's Health (NCCWHC). (2007). *Intrapartum care. Care of healthy women and their babies during childbirth. Clinical guideline*. London: RCOG.

NHS Litigation Authority. (2009a). *CNST maternity clinical risk management standards*. London: NHSLA.

NHS Litigation Authority. (2009b). *Study of stillbirth claims*. London: NHSLA.

O'Connor, M C, Hassabo, M S, & McFadyen, R. (1980). Is the sinusoidal fetal heart rate pattern sinister? *Journal of Obstetrics and Gynaecology, 1*, 90–95.

Samueloff, A., Langer, O., & Berkus, M. (1994). Is fetal heart rate variability a good predictor of fetal outcome. *Acta Obstetrica and Gynecologica Scandanavica, 73*, 39–44.

Schneider, E. P., & Tropper, P. J. (1986). Variable deceleration, prolonged deceleration and sinusoidal fetal heart rate. *Clinical Obstetrics and Gynaecology, 29*, 64–72.

Serra, V., Bellver, J., & Moulden, N., et al. (2009). Computerized analysis of normal fetal heart rate pattern throughout gestation. *Ultrasound in Obstetrics and Gynaecology, 34*, 74–79.

Spencer, JA, & Johnson, P. (1986). Fetal heart rate variability changes and fetal behavioural cycles during labour. *British Journal of Obstetrics and Gynaecology, 93*, 314–321.

Litigation and the CTG

Andrew Symon

PART 3

INTRODUCTION

DISCLAIMER

Although electronic fetal monitoring has featured in litigation (otherwise why have this chapter?), litigation should be at the back of your mind when you use this technology. There are good clinical reasons for using CTGs. Litigation, or the fear of it, is not a valid reason.

In Part 1 of this book, the indications for electronic fetal monitoring (EFM) were described, and the reader will by now have a good appreciation of the when/why/how of this. Part 2 dealt with the interpretation of cardiotocograph (CTG) traces, and now Part 3 examines the role played by cardiotocography in litigation, mostly involving allegations of clinical negligence. Part 3 will show how debates about CTG use and its interpretation are sometimes critical when the clinical outcome is poor, and legal action ensues. The main section of this part will refer to legal cases when examining 'When to monitor?', 'Difficulties with monitoring', 'Using the equipment correctly', 'Interpretation of the trace', 'Delay in responding', and 'Staying up to date'. There's also a final section called 'Some reassuring news'.

It is beyond the scope of this part to discuss the rights and wrongs of the current legal position, where blame must be established in order to secure financial compensation. Neither will it explore the possible motives behind litigation, or the likelihood of success when people do sue. Those wishing to learn more about the law of medical negligence generally are referred to standard texts (Dimond 2006; Mason and Laurie 2010); time factors and success rates in cerebral palsy litigation are discussed by Symon (2002); success rates in obstetric litigation generally are discussed by Symon (2001) and NHS Litigation Authority (2010).

It is sufficient for our purposes to restate the basic tenet of clinical negligence litigation, which is that in order to establish negligence, a plaintiff ('pursuer' in Scotland) has to satisfy three tests:

1. that there was a duty of care (this is rarely in doubt)
2. that this duty of care was breached (the standard of care must be examined in order to demonstrate this)
3. that the breach of the duty of care caused or materially contributed to the damage.

Cerebral palsy claims often revolve around the second and third of these tests, but this chapter will focus principally on the second (standard of care) test, since this is of most direct importance to clinical practitioners.

Because the full clinical picture of cerebral palsy does not always manifest immediately, legal claims often take many years to come to light, and, unlike other clinical negligence actions, there is effectively no time limit in which a claim must be brought. Memory recall after several months can be problematic. After several years it is usually absent, and so clinical documentation is relied upon to establish the relevant facts. Gibb and Arulkumaran (2007) note: 'The importance of careful, legible note keeping is obvious. Regrettably, in many hospitals the standard is poor.'

BACKGROUND TO CTG LITIGATION

Obstetric litigation (which includes allegations against midwives) is high-profile in litigation terms. It is not the most common clinical specialty for legal cases in the UK (surgery enjoys that dubious distinction), but the potential for large compensation payouts makes it by far the most expensive (NHS Litigation Authority 2010). The reason for this is the huge amounts which are required for the lifelong care of someone who has suffered irreversible cerebral damage. While obstetric litigation is high-profile, the likelihood of any one midwife being involved is still low, certainly beyond the report-writing stage.

As noted in Part 1, continuous EFM was introduced in the 1970s with the hope that it would reduce the incidence of cerebral palsy, but although the caesarean rate has increased hugely in that time, cerebral palsy rates have remained more or less static. The American College of Obstetricians and Gynecologists (2009) has acknowledged that 'the false-positive rate of electronic fetal monitoring (EFM) for predicting cerebral palsy is high, at greater than 99%'. The 2009 American College of Obstetricians and Gynecologists guidelines have seen the 'reassuring/non-reassuring' categorisation of traces replaced with 'normal/intermediate/abnormal', a move which Dickens and Cook (2010) believe is likely 'to reduce the risk of … over-reacting to FHR [fetal heart rate] traces, and precipitately urging and undertaking cesarean deliveries'. However, the limitations of EFM and the growing awareness that only a small minority of cases of cerebral palsy can be attributed to an intrapartum insult have not yet reduced the focus on CTG use during labour. Indeed the National Institute for Health and Clinical Excellence (NICE) (2007) guidelines on intrapartum care make specific recommendations on when to use EFM. The purpose of this chapter is to highlight some of the areas of vulnerability for practitioners when they use the CTG.

Increased CTG use has been cited as an example of defensive clinical practice (Symon 2000, 2001; Greer 2010) – where clinical procedures are undertaken or avoided because of a fear of legal consequences. Practitioners should be wary of adopting such an approach, not least because it may be clinically counterproductive. Graham et al. (2006) note that 'meta-analysis of the randomized controlled trials comparing EFM with auscultation have found an increased incidence of cesarean delivery and decreased neonatal seizures, but no effect on the incidence of cerebral palsy or perinatal death'. Also in the USA, Miller and Depp (2008) note that 'EFM is another intervention intended to improve pregnancy outcomes that has been widely integrated into standard obstetric practice without yielding any evidence to support a reduction in cerebral palsy following term deliveries or otherwise'.

EFM clearly has limitations, and so it must be used with caution, and interpreted carefully. The lack of a general appreciation of these limitations is lamented by Hankins et al. (2006): 'many judges, jurors and plaintiffs in cerebral palsy lawsuits appear to be unaware of the fallibility of the high-tech gadgetry of modern obstetrics, including EFM, and that these devices cannot reliably predict or influence obstetric outcome'. They were referring to the situation in the USA, and while there are many similarities between the USA and the UK, we must be cautious about extrapolating from American studies. For example, juries are not used in negligence cases in the UK, and the majority of US compensation awards apparently goes towards legal fees and administrative costs (Hankins et al. 2006). Nevertheless, there are some similarities in terms of cerebral palsy litigation: it often concerns absent or inadequate EFM, a slow response to a poor trace and the claim that a birth was not effected quickly enough. Clark et al. (2008) found that 'delayed physician evaluation of a non-reassuring fetal heart rate tracing and delayed delivery' were significant features in their study of closed American legal claims.

Litigation concerning cerebral palsy is often initiated many years after the birth in question (see the note above about memory recall). This does not reduce the level of distress for all concerned. One thing to bear in mind is that the standards applied to judge whether practitioners acted appropriately or not are those standards which were current at the time. In other words, developments in the understanding of the fetal heart rate, or changes in accepted practice since the birth, will be disregarded. However, it is now recognised that 'system errors' as well as individual mistakes may contribute to a poor clinical outcome. Miller (2005) makes the point that 'even the most well-educated clinician will be set up to fail if operating in a system where communication is problematic'. Some acknowledgement may be given of this concerning cases originating years ago, even though that awareness was not around at the time in question.

THE CTG IN LITIGATION

In the early 1990s there was a flurry of interest in obstetric litigation. Ennis and Vincent (1990) identified allegations concerning unsatisfactory or missing traces, abnormalities being ignored or not noticed, and traces simply not being done. Of 11 in this category, they note that in three 'midwives were asked by a doctor to carry out CTG but forgot'. The problem of a CTG trace going missing was also noted by James (1991): 'The cardiotocograph record is often crucial yet its bulk at the end of a long and complicated labour makes it difficult to store securely within the records. However, claims have become indefensible because this vital piece of evidence was missing, the notes were inadequate, or key personnel could not be traced'.

Capstick and Edwards (1990) identified problems with not noticing signs of fetal distress, or not taking appropriate action quickly when such signs were noticed. Vincent et al. (1991) noted that missing or poor-quality traces were significant, and also found that interpretation was a recurrent theme: 'In 14 cases the doctor or midwife simply did not recognise an abnormal trace. In five the abnormality was noted, but no action was taken; the staff believed the machine to be faulty and so ignored the trace.'

These somewhat dated references prompted a debate about clinical practice, and about the efficiency of the legal system when dealing with medical negligence claims. Concerns about the expense of litigation (and obstetric litigation in particular) led to suggestions that no-fault schemes and structured settlements should be introduced, along with greater use of alternative methods of dispute resolution, such as mediation. A report by the Lord Chancellor (Lord Chancellor's Department 2002) highlighted the political desire for reform: litigation was to be avoided where possible, and it was to be less complex and less adversarial when it did occur. Litigation concerning CTG interpretation was an integral part of this debate.

The initial concerns about CTGs in the early 1990s highlighted a number of deficiencies in their use. It would be hoped that this awareness would lead to improvements in the following years. However, the legal cases described here, which extend from the mid-1990s to the present day, illustrate that practitioners continue to be found wanting at times. The extracts include allegations of failing to use the CTG when there was an indication to do so, the inappropriate use of equipment and poor interpretation of the CTG trace. These extracts are merely illustrative, and the success (or otherwise) of these cases should not be inferred from the details given.

Some of the cases are from my own doctoral research in the 1990s (these have been anonymised, and are referred to simply as Case 1, Case 2, etc.) and others are from publicly reported court cases (the vast majority of legal actions do not get as far as the court stage). Citations for the court cases are given, and although the judgement transcripts are public documents I have used pseudonyms for the clinical staff: their identities are not important for the lessons outlined here, and their involvement in litigation will have been stressful enough. Intrapartum care is multidisciplinary where the CTG is concerned, and so these cases concern both midwives and obstetricians.

When to monitor?

In Part 1 the indications for EFM were discussed. Guidelines about this came about in part because of failures to monitor when it was apparent that this should have happened.

In one of the cases reviewed, there were persistent early fetal heart rate decelerations. The midwifery staff appeared to think these were benign, despite there being reduced fetal heart rate variability and meconium staining of the liquor. The expert report stated:

> *Case 1 There is a period of 90 minutes ... when there was no CTG recording. This is an unacceptable situation where the patient has had a previous section, [is] at 42 weeks with meconium staining, and with CTG abnormalities which are persistent and who was on oxytocin.*

This catalogue of 'at-risk' factors does not appear to have alerted midwives to the need for extra vigilance, and, unsurprisingly, this case was conceded by the defence. However, given the desire of some pregnant women for minimal monitoring and intervention in labour, the decision to use the CTG is not always automatic, even when certain 'at-risk' factors are present (for a discussion of the risk–choice paradox, see Symon 2006). In another case the woman complained that she should have been monitored more closely, despite having asked in advance of her labour for minimal monitoring. In fact during labour the CTG had been discontinued at her request due to discomfort. Her solicitor claimed:

> *Case 2 Continuous fetal monitoring when the decision was made to give a Syntocinon infusion should have been insisted upon...*

This case illustrates the balancing act which staff must attempt when responding to a specific request, while using clinical judgement and (increasingly) deciding whether to follow unit protocols which may contradict the woman's stated preference. Sadly, cases involving the use (and misuse) of Syntocinon are not rare. In addition to careful monitoring (NICE 2007) and sympathetic care, midwives must keep meticulous notes in such a situation, including a full account of the nature of the uterine contractions. Because of synthetic oxytocin's known potential for causing uterine hyperstimulation and consequent fetal compromise, extreme care must be taken when using it. In one Irish case the judge noted:

> *I find on the evidence that Senior Midwife Collins was negligent and in breach of duty in not calling Dr. Smith at 06:50 hours and in not turning off the oxytocin and ... was further guilty of negligence and breach of duty in failing to call Dr. Smith at between 07:10 hours and 07:12 hours* (Fitzpatrick v National Maternity Hospital *[2008]; per Herbert J).*

The difficulties of determining the level of uterine activity when Syntocinon is used were well expressed in another case (*L v Royal Victoria Infirmary* [2005]):

> *The first point on which [the obstetric experts] disagree is whether there is, as a matter of fact, sufficient evidence of hyperstimulation following the increase in Syntocinon at 17:48 hrs. Mr Johnson in a tabular chronology identified raised baseline pressure on the CTG at 18:00, definite hyperstimulation at 18:40, and what he called instances of uterine irritability at 19:10 and 19:45. I have to say that, in accordance with Professor Thornton's view, I am unable to discern any significant changes on the trace at any of these times other than 18:40, particularly in view of the accepted limitations of monitoring by an external transducer (per Langan J @ 75).*

The bottom line is that particular care must be taken whenever Syntocinon is in use. While it is accepted that there are times when effective monitoring is difficult to achieve, the importance of documentation cannot be overstated.

Difficulties with monitoring

Midwives have sometimes found it difficult to monitor effectively:

> *Case 3 The plaintiffs claimed that monitoring should not have been discontinued. The midwife documented that it was very difficult to listen to the fetal heart as the labouring woman moved and rocked a lot.*
>
> *The midwife looking after her noted frequent 'loss of contact' on the CTG trace, and stated: 'I made the decision to stop the printout from the monitor but kept the transducer and belt in situ, and I was continually listening to the fetal heart.'*

The midwives' reports indicated that the fetal heart rate was satisfactory at all times, but there is clearly a difficulty in situations like this. When a probe must be held in position in order to hear the fetal heart rate clearly, writing contemporaneous entries in the woman's case notes is impossible. In another case the midwife stated:

> *Case 4 As I was anxious to get a better-quality CTG, I didn't take my hands off the transducer and was aware that I wasn't recording this in the case notes.*

The midwife must be able to ensure several things at once: in addition to providing clinical care, she must make sure that a reasonable CTG trace is produced, and that she completes the clinical notes as soon as she can.

In another case (*Azzam v The General Medical Council* [2008]), which related to fitness to practise and not alleged negligence, the judge noted:

> *The oxytocin was increased every 15 minutes. At its increase in rate at 15:30 Midwife Callaghan had recorded that she was having strong urges to push and that the contractions were 3–4 every 10 minutes. On the CTG there is no contraction belt recording present at this stage … While between 15:30 and 15:50 the CTG is difficult to interpret, it does appear that she is getting deep decelerations but because there is a non-recording of the contractions it is difficult to tell whether these are variable or late decelerations (per McCombe J @4).*

The CTG tracing must be of sufficient quality that others can interpret it. Williams and Arulkumaran (2004) note: 'The courts will view an uninterpretable CTG with utmost suspicion and such a recording might jeopardise a successful defence.'

Using the equipment correctly

In another legal case the plaintiff's solicitors claimed:

> *Case 5 It would appear that a fetal monitor was incorrectly adjusted and, accordingly, the readings which it gave were not properly interpreted and significant abnormalities were disregarded.*

The CTG had 'wrong speed' written on it. It transpired that different speeds were used at different times in labour, and no times were logged, so the trace was more difficult to interpret. (The case occurred a number of years ago; contemporary CTG machines automatically print the date and time on the trace regularly.)

There have been times when the CTG machine itself appears to cause problems:

> *Case 6 The plaintiff's solicitors claimed that, instead of diagnosing fetal distress in labour, staff assumed the 'heart rate coming and going' was due to a defective CTG machine. Only when the third machine (they claim) was showing the same sort of trace was the woman sent for caesarean section.*
>
> *There was nothing documented to say the CTG machine was replaced at all. Eventually the CTG traces were found, and they revealed one change of machine, from an old to a new model.*

The fact that equipment is defective is no defence. In this case there was a gap of 2½ hours when the CTG was not on. There were six written recordings of a fetal heart rate during this period, at half-hourly intervals. The expert report criticised the midwives for not having a more detailed record.

A simple, and yet vital, part of the CTG machine is the clock. In *CJL v West Midlands Strategic Health Authority* [2009] the judge noted:

> *It is common ground that the time 22:06 is the time according to the machine's clock. But the clock cannot have been correctly set, because the printed times are one hour later than the times handwritten on the same part of the roll as that on which the printed time appears. It is common ground that where it records 22:06, then that is to be read as 21:06. Presumably the machine had not been reset for daylight saving time (per Tugendhat J @ 14).*

This is embarrassing, but easily explained. In fact this case turned on a specific 2-minute period. Where the CTG and wall clocks are just a few minutes apart it can make determining the sequence of events problematic. This in turn can make it difficult to justify a practitioner's actions.

Interpretation of the trace

It seems obvious that staff who use CTGs must be able to interpret them, but sadly this ability is lacking all too often. Williams and Arulkumaran (2004) claim that 'CTG misinterpretation is the most common source of alleged negligence in obstetric litigation and the inexact nature of CTG traces causes great confusion in court'. The recent American College of Obstetricians and Gynecologists guideline (2009) noted that 'there is high interobserver and intraobserver variability in interpretation of FHR tracing'.

In an Irish case (*Fitzpatrick v National Maternity Hospital* [2008]) the judge noted:

> *The issue of negligence centred principally on the claim that the [staff] failed to properly interpret the cardiotocograph record … and failed to act correctly in the light of that record … I find on the evidence that by 07:12 hours it must have been very obvious to Senior Midwife Collins that a pattern of very deep decelerations with no baseline variability was established … Even faced with this emergency, Senior Midwife Collins still did not summon Dr. Smith (per Herbert J).*

Even seniority in this case did not protect the midwife from severe criticism.

Sometimes the criticism is of several staff, as in *Lowe v. Yorkhill NHS Trust* [2007]:

> *Taken broadly, it was argued on behalf of the pursuer that the medical and midwifery staff responsible for Mrs Lowe's care had been negligent in failing to appreciate the significance of the CTG readings available from 08:21 onwards. It was said that had they properly interpreted the information available to them an assisted delivery would have been performed at an earlier stage, thus avoiding the subsequent circulatory collapse and brain injury (per Lord Turnbull @ 11).*

Just because an allegation such as this is made, it does not necessarily follow that it is true. While this may be little comfort for practitioners dragged through the litigation process, the final outcome ought to bring some relief. However, there are times when it is very hard to understand the inactivity of the staff. In one case the expert report stated:

> *Case 7 I do not recall having ever seen a trace with such a smooth line and almost complete lack of beat to beat variation … The nursing [sic] staff faithfully recorded the events but apparently failed to appreciate the significance of the flat trace and therefore did not report it to the medical staff.*

There are other cases in which the CTG has shown abnormalities which were ignored by staff. In one instance the expert reported:

> *Case 8 It is difficult to see the point of fetal monitoring if no action is to be taken when there are obvious abnormalities in the recording.*

Staff must be educated and trained in order to make an intelligent interpretation of CTG traces. However, all too frequently it must be questioned whether staff are adequately prepared for this part of their work. In another case a junior midwife was heavily criticised by the defence solicitor:

> *Case 9 [The midwife] admitted quite freely that she spent many hours in watching a fetal heart monitor which she was insufficiently trained to interpret or understand at the time. She has since been better trained and, looking back at the fetal heart traces during the period she was on duty, she sees them as being abnormal. In my opinion, quite a bit of liability must therefore attach to a system which asked midwives to watch a monitor which they are insufficiently trained to understand.*

All staff, of whatever grade, must be trained in CTG interpretation if they are called upon to use the technology, and compliance with risk management standards now includes mandatory training for the relevant staff.

One of the crucial aspects of CTG interpretation is that it is not an exact science – even experts will disagree at times, as noted in *Lowe v Yorkhill NHS Trust* [2007]:

> *His description of the decelerations which preceded the prolonged deceleration at 08:47 differed from that given by Dr Milne. Whereas Dr Milne had described these as being mostly of the late variety, Dr Smith termed them as variable or atypical variable decelerations. However he was keen to make the point that one ought not to categorise a trace by looking at a single deceleration. One ought to take a group of about five to ten together and arrive at a categorisation (per Lord Turnbull @ 36).*

The Dr C Bravado mnemonic (determine risk; contractions; baseline rate; variability; accelerations; decelerations; overall assessment) makes it clear that the overall picture must be taken into account, and not just isolated parts of a CTG trace.

The quotation above in the 'When to monitor?' section (*L v Royal Victoria Infirmary* [2005]) also makes the point that senior practitioners disagree on occasion. Sadly, it is sometimes the midwife who is seen to have failed to recognise and deal with a problem. In *Khalid v Barnet & Chase Farm Hospital* [2007] the judge referred to:

> *the period following 06:15 when it is agreed Midwife Thomson should have called Dr Carr, the obstetric registrar on duty that night, as a result of the CTG becoming what is termed 'pathological' … At 06:15 there were early decelerations down to 80 [baseline 160]. The experts agree in their joint statement that the midwife at this stage (06:15/20) should have called for medical assistance because of the persistent tachycardia and variable decelerations (per Judge Grenfell @ 20 and 28).*

Inevitably, failing to recognise a problem, and thereafter to deal with it, leads to delay in appropriate management. The next section now takes this up.

Delay in responding

A delay in appropriate management may result either from non-recognition of an abnormal trace, or inaction following the diagnosis of such an abnormality. Appropriate action may be to 'wait and see' for a limited period (e.g. while the Syntocinon infusion is reduced or discontinued, or maternal hydration carried out) but this must be explained fully in the notes. Williams and Arulkumaran (2004) state: 'Initialling the CTG is not enough'.

Ennis and Vincent (1990) report that in some of the legal cases they analysed midwives had correctly noted a fetal heart rate abnormality, but this was ignored by the doctor. As noted above, differences of opinion do occur. Such differences were highlighted in related research (Symon 1998) which examined the views of a large number of midwives and obstetricians concerning litigation and certain related aspects. In this research one doctor commented that:

> *Overdiagnosis of 'distress' is a large problem.*

From the midwife's point of view there came this comment:

> *It can be very frustrating for midwives to inform doctors of a suspected abnormality, to have it ignored before client, and to have to repeatedly call the doctor back.*

In the *Azzam* case, such a difference of opinion was reported:

> *The evidence showed that at 16:15 hours Dr Azzam had been called to the mother's room by the midwife who was having difficulty in interpreting the CTG trace. The witnesses said that Dr Azzam only scanned the trace cursorily, perhaps for about 25 seconds. The expert evidence was that this examination of the trace was inadequate and that about a minute at least would be required by a careful doctor to interpret the trace satisfactorily (per McCombe J @ 5).*

Such differences of opinion must be addressed, and it is one of the aims of risk management to do this. However, it is more concerning when a midwife fails to take appropriate steps to call in more senior colleagues, as in this case in which a consultant obstetrician reported:

> *Case 10 There is little doubt that at 23:30 hours acute profound fetal bradycardia occurred and the delay of 20 minutes before medical assistance was summoned is indefensible ... Equally it seems that the outcome was not helped by the 6-minute interval between delivery and the arrival of the paediatrician ... What ... is inexcusable is that he was not summoned prior to the delivery given the circumstances of this profound and protracted bradycardia in the last half-hour of labour.*

Maternity care is multidisciplinary, and midwives must appreciate the respective roles of other practitioners, and involve them appropriately.

In the *Khalid v Barnet & Chase Farm Hospital* [2007] case noted above, the judge was critical of the midwife and her delay in acting appropriately, and in his summing up stated that this delay had been critical:

> *I am satisfied that it is more likely than not that the operation would have taken place more than 20 minutes earlier than it did; that, therefore, this breach of duty caused the operation to take place 20 minutes later than it should have taken place and [the baby] to suffer damage that [she] would not otherwise have suffered (per Grenfell J @ 95).*

Staying up to date

As noted above, compliance with risk management standards means that staff who use the CTG must receive regular updates. Practices and guidelines do change over time as more becomes known about the significance of CTG interpretations. Practitioners should remember that they cannot be judged by knowledge that only became available after the events in question.

That it is tempting to use information that has become available was acknowledged by Lord Turnbull in *Lowe v Yorkhill NHS Trust* [2007].

> *In common with all of the other relevant witnesses Midwife Jones was examined at length on the contents of the NICE Guidelines. However, these guidelines were not issued until May 2001, more than two years after the birth of [the baby] (@ 18).*

Only the accepted practice or understanding of the day can be used to judge whether a practitioner's actions were appropriate or not. Not staying up to date would be looked upon gravely.

Some reassuring news

This discussion of legal cases may give the impression that litigation is commonplace, and that practitioners will be put through the mill. There is no doubt that being involved in litigation is extremely stressful, but I repeat the fact that it is still rare for midwives to become involved, certainly beyond the 'writing a report' stage.

It is also the case that good practice is a safeguard, both against being involved in litigation, and against being found to have been negligent. One such practice involves writing relevant information on the CTG trace, and in one case (*Beasley v Fife Health Board* [2001]) this was held to have been critical:

> *The pursuer's evidence is quite clear. She said she never changed position and her feet never left the bed. She denied her legs were moved. It has to be remembered that she was in agony at childbirth and her evidence about changes in position is contradicted by the CTG entries which are deemed to be accurate (per Lord McEwan @ 84).*

So, good practice can save your skin.

CONCLUSION

All the suggestions and comments made in this chapter may seem obvious. However, if the problems caused by failing to implement these points were rare, they would not be cited here. Many poor outcomes (and subsequent legal cases) simply would not arise if these points were taken on board and implemented effectively. It is disheartening to realise that certain errors continue to be made despite a recognition that they can often be prevented. However, we don't live in an ideal world: staff will have 'off days', communication with colleagues and with women and their families may be difficult, and pressure of work may leave little time for contemporaneous documentation.

CTGs, however, remain a critical part of intrapartum care in high-risk cases, and constitute a significant factor in litigation. Risk management in this respect is the responsibility of both employers and of individual practitioners.

REFERENCES

American College of Obstetricians and Gynecologists. (2009). *Intrapartum fetal heart rate monitoring: Nomenclature, interpretation, and general management principles* (pp. 2, 8). Washington (DC): ACOG. (ACOG practice bulletin; no. 106).

Capstick, J. B., & Edwards, P. (1990). Trends in obstetric malpractice claims. *Lancet, 336*, 931–932.

Clark, S. L., Belfort, M. A., & Dildy, G. A., et al. (2008). Reducing obstetric litigation through alterations in practice patterns. *Obstetrics and Gynecology, 112*, 1279–1283.

Dickens, B. M., & Cook, R. J. (2010). The legal effects of fetal monitoring guidelines. *International Journal of Gynecology & Obstetrics, 108*, 170–173.

Dimond, B. (2006). *The legal aspects of midwifery* (3rd ed.). Edinburgh: Elsevier (Books for Midwives Press).

Ennis, M., & Vincent, C. A. (1990). Obstetric accidents: a review of 64 cases. *British Medical Journal, 300*, 1365–1367.

Gibb, D., & Arulkumaran, S. (2007). *Fetal monitoring in practice* (3rd ed., p. 227). Edinburgh: Churchill Livingstone.

Graham, E. M., Petersen, S. M., & Christo, D. K., et al. (2006). Intrapartum electronic fetal heart rate monitoring and the prevention of perinatal brain injury. *Obstetrics and Gynecology, 108*, 656–666.

Greer, J. (2010). Are midwives irrational or afraid? *Evidence-Based Midwifery, 8*, 47–52.

Hankins, G. D. V., MacLennan, A. H., & Speer, M. E. (2006). Obstetric litigation is asphyxiating our maternity services. *Obstetrics & Gynecology, 107*, 1382–1385.

James, C. (1991). Risk management in obstetrics and gynaecology. *Journal of the Medical Defence Union, 7*, 36–38.

Lord Chancellor's Department, *Civil justice evaluation: Further findings*. The Lord Chancellor's Department. (Online. Available at: <http://www.dca.gov.uk/civil/reform/ffreform.htm>)

Mason, J. K., & Laurie, G. T. (2010). *Mason and McCall Smith's law and medical ethics* (8th ed.). Oxford: OUP.

Miller, L. A. (2005). System errors in intrapartum electronic fetal monitoring: A case review. *Journal of Midwifery and Women's Health, 50*, 507–516.

Miller, R., & Depp, R. (2008). Minimizing perinatal neurologic injury at term: Is cesarean section the answer? *Clinics in Perinatology, 35*, 549–559.

National Institute for Health and Clinical Excellence (NICE). (2007). *Intrapartum care: Care of healthy women and their babies during childbirth*. Clinical Guideline 55, revised 2008. London: RCOG, National Collaborating Centre for Women's and Children's Health.

NHS Litigation Authority. (2010). *The NHS litigation authority factsheet 3: Information on claims*. London: NHSLA. (see 'Publications/NHSLA Factsheets in <http://www.nhsla.com>)

Symon, A. (1998). *Who's accountable? Who's to blame? Litigation - the views of midwives and obstetricians*. Hale: Hochland and Hochland.

Symon, A. (2000). Litigation and defensive clinical practice: Quantifying the problem. *Midwifery, 16*, 8–14.

Symon, A. (2001). *Obstetric Litigation from A-Z*. Salisbury: Quay Books.

Symon, A. (2002). The significance of time factors in cerebral palsy litigation. *Midwifery, 18*, 35–42.

Symon, A. (2006). Risk and choice in maternity care. In A. Symon (Ed.), *The risk–choice paradox*. Edinburgh: Elsevier.

Vincent, C., Martin, T., & Ennis, M. (1991). Obstetric accidents: the patient's perspective. *British Journal of Obstetrics & Gynaecology, 98*, 390–395.

Williams, B., & Arulkumaran, S. (2004). Cardiotocography and medicolegal issues. *Best Practice & Research: Clinical Obstetrics & Gynaecology, 18*, 457–466.

PUBLISHED LEGAL CASES CITED IN THIS CHAPTER

Azzam v The General Medical Council. (2008). EWHC 2711 (Admin).

Beasley (AP) v Fife Health Board. (2001). Scot CS 229.

CJL (a child) v West Midlands Strategic Health Authority. (2009). EWHC 259 (QB).

Fitzpatrick [a minor] v National Maternity Hospital. (2008). IEHC 62.

Khalid (a child) v Barnet & Chase Farm Hospital NHS Trust. (2007). EWHC 644 (QB).

L (a child) v Royal Victoria Infirmary and Associated Hospitals NHS Trust. (2005). EWHC B4 (QB).

Lowe v Yorkhill NHS Trust. (2007). Scot CS CSOH 111.

Case Studies

CONTENTS

PART **4**

Normal

SECTION 1

Fig. 4.1

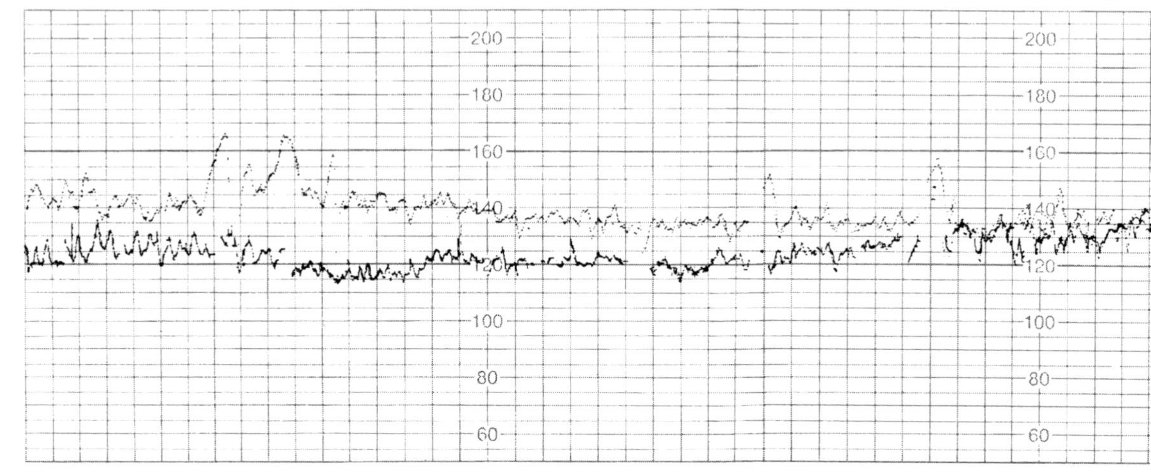

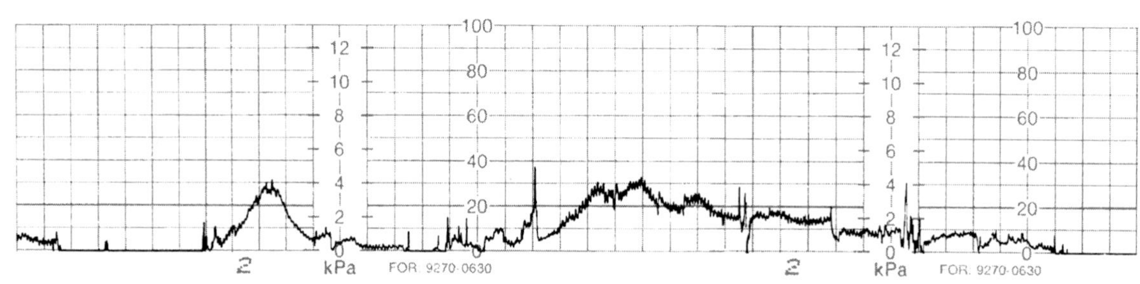

HISTORY

25-year-old gravida 3, para 1 + 1.

Past history

Nil relevant.

Antenatal period

Twin pregnancy diagnosed on booking scan. Admitted at 37 weeks with spontaneous rupture of membranes and contractions.

Labour

04.00 hours

Cervical os 4 cm dilated.
Clear liquor draining.
Fetal scalp electrode applied to twin 1 (faint line on CTG).
Twin 2 monitored externally (darker line on CTG).
Contractions monitored externally.

04.50 hours

Epidural analgesia commenced.

06.00 hours

Cervical os 6 cm dilated.
CTG (Fig. 4.1).

CTG

1 What do you notice about the baseline?
2 What do you notice about the baseline variability?
3 What periodic changes, if any, are present?
4 What do you notice about the uterine activity?
5 Would you categorise this CTG as normal/suspicious/pathological?
6 What is the most probable cause of fetal heart rate abnormality shown on this trace?
7 What treatment and/or intervention would you consider necessary for this fetal heart rate pattern?

NOTES

1

2

3

4

5

6

7

ANALYSIS

Twin 1 (dark line)

1	Baseline 135–140 bpm	**Reassuring**
2	Variability 5–10 beats	**Reassuring**
3	Accelerations present	**Reassuring**
	No decelerations	**Reassuring**

Twin 2 (faint line)

Baseline 115–120 bpm	**Reassuring**
Variability 5–10 beats	**Reassuring**
Accelerations present	**Reassuring**
No decelerations	**Reassuring**

4 Contractions not monitored adequately.

5 All features fall into reassuring category: the CTG is classified as normal.

6 No abnormalities present.

7 Contractions should be monitored. No other action is necessary. When monitoring the fetal heart rate of twins there can be difficulties in interpretation if the fetal heart rates are very similar. Most modern monitors now allow for the fetal heart rates to be recorded with a 20-beat difference for a 10-minute period. This allows for clearer interpretation.

OUTCOME

10.35 hours

Progressed to second stage of labour.

12.06 hours

Straight forceps delivery of twin 1.
Live girl.
Apgar score 9/1 9/5.
Birthweight 2.470 kg.

12.20 hours

Straight forceps delivery of twin 2.
Live girl.
Apgar score 8/1 9/5. Birthweight 2.560 kg.

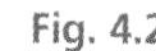
Fig. 4.2

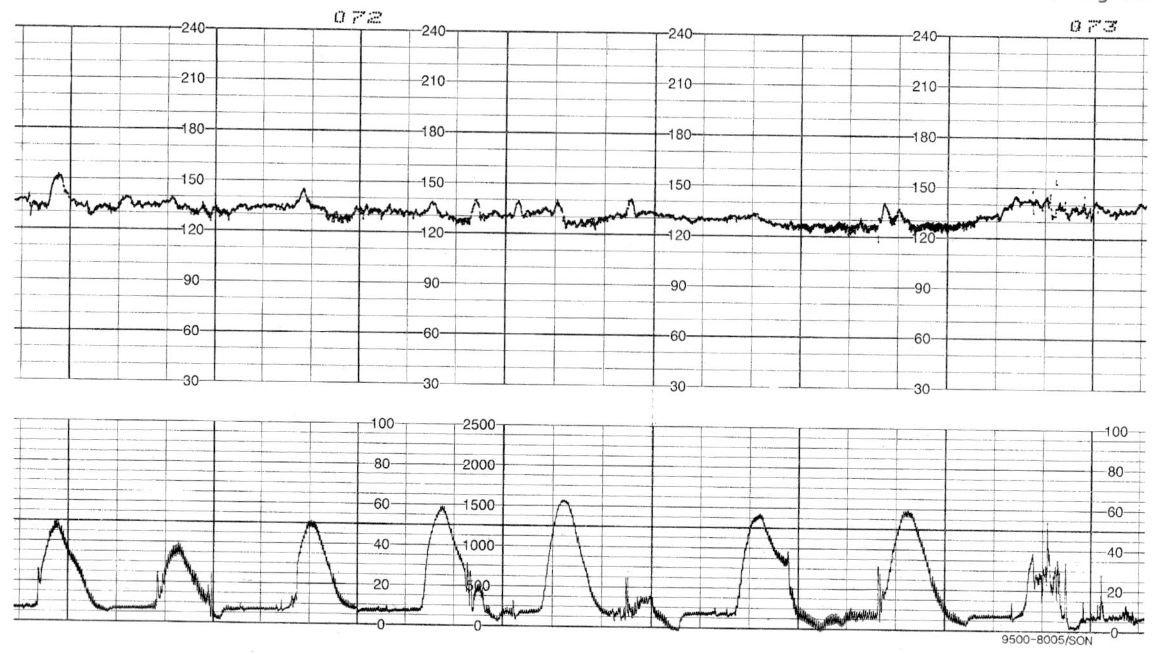

HISTORY

30-year-old gravida 2, para 1.

Past history

Nil relevant.

Antenatal period

Progressed normally.
Admitted at 41 + 2 in spontaneous labour.

Labour

03.20 hours

Cervical os 7 cm dilated.
Clear liquor draining.
Requesting epidural analgesia.

03.40 hours

Epidural analgesia commenced.
Continuous external monitoring in progress.

04.30 hours

CTG (Fig. 4.2).

CTG

1. What do you notice about the baseline?
2. What do you notice about the baseline variability?
3. What periodic changes, if any, are present?
4. What do you notice about the uterine activity?
5. Would you categorise this CTG as normal/suspicious/pathological?
6. What is the most probable cause of fetal heart rate abnormality shown on this trace?
7. What treatment and/or intervention would you consider necessary for this fetal heart rate pattern?

NOTES

1

2

3

4

5

6

7

ANALYSIS

1	Baseline 130–135 bpm	**Reassuring**
2	Variability around 5 beats	**Reassuring**
3	No decelerations, accelerations present	**Reassuring**
4	Contracting 3–4 in 10 minutes.	
5	All features reassuring: CTG classified as normal.	
6	No abnormalities present.	
7	No action necessary.	

OUTCOME

Progressed to second stage of labour.

09.58 hours

Normal delivery.
Live boy.
Apgar score 9/1 9/5.
Birthweight 3.58 kg.

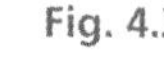

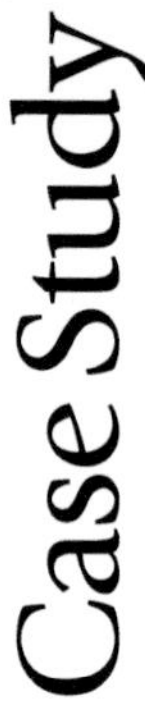

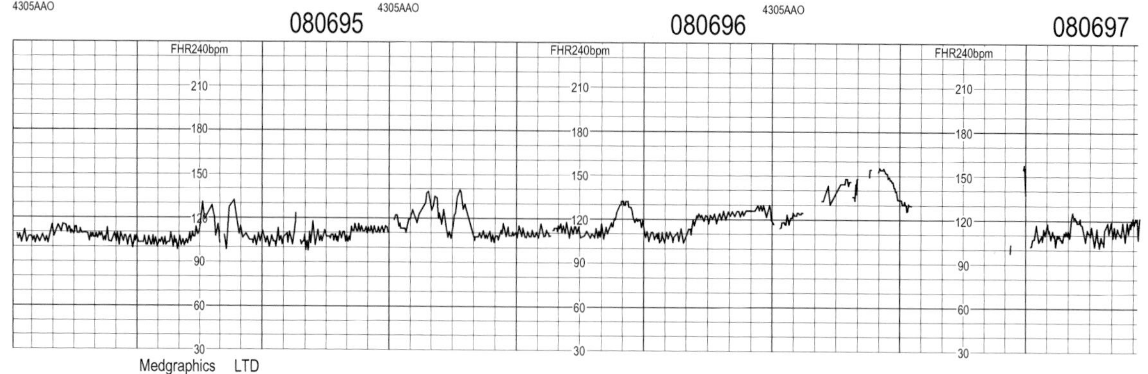

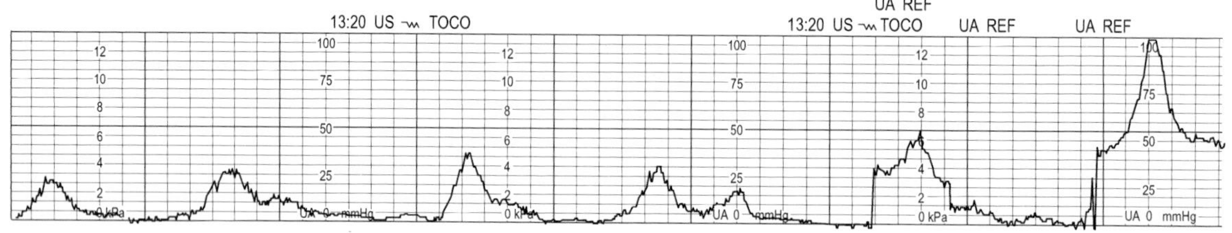

Fig. 4.3

HISTORY

24-year-old gravida 4, para 1 + 2.

Past history

Previous normal delivery.
Deep-vein thrombosis 6 years ago, on Fragmin (dalteparin sodium).

Antenatal period

Normal.
Admitted at 39 weeks' gestation in spontaneous labour.

Labour

Vaginal assessment on admission revealed cervix to be thin and well applied to presenting part; cervical os was 5 cm dilated.
Membranes intact.
Fetal heart monitored by external transducer.
No analgesia.
CTG (Fig. 4.3).

CTG

1 What do you notice about the baseline?
2 What do you notice about the baseline variability?
3 What periodic changes, if any, are present?
4 What do you notice about the uterine activity?
5 Would you categorise this CTG as normal/suspicious/pathological?
6 What is the most probable cause of fetal heart rate abnormality shown on this trace?
7 What treatment and/or intervention would you consider necessary for this fetal heart rate pattern?

NOTES

1

2

3

4

5

6

7

ANALYSIS

1 Baseline 110 bpm — **Reassuring**
2 Variability 5–10 beats — **Reassuring**
3 None, accelerations with contractions — **Reassuring**
4 Contracting 1:3.
5 All features reassuring: CTG classifies as normal.
6 No abnormalities.
7 No action required. This woman has been deemed as low-risk during labour. Intermittent auscultation is the recommended method of fetal heart rate monitoring. The reason for continuous fetal heart rate monitoring in labour should be questioned. Following discussion between the woman and her midwife, highlighting best-practice guidelines, intermittent auscultation should be offered as the preferred method of fetal heart rate monitoring. If the woman chooses continuous monitoring there must be documentary evidence in the case notes of the risks and benefits that were discussed and that informed consent was gained.

OUTCOME

At the end of the portion of CTG, the woman was feeling urges to push. A repeat vaginal assessment revealed the cervix to be thin and well applied to the presenting part. The cervical os was 9 cm dilated. Membranes were ruptured artificially with clear liquor evident.
The CTG remained in progress.

Second stage of labour was diagnosed 15 minutes later. Progress was slow, resulting in a straight forceps delivery 2 hours into the second stage.
Live girl, Apgar score 8 and 8. Birthweight 3.260 kg.

Cord gases	pH	Base excess (mmol/l)
UA	7.13	5.5
UV	7.27	6.5

Fig. 4.4, Part 1

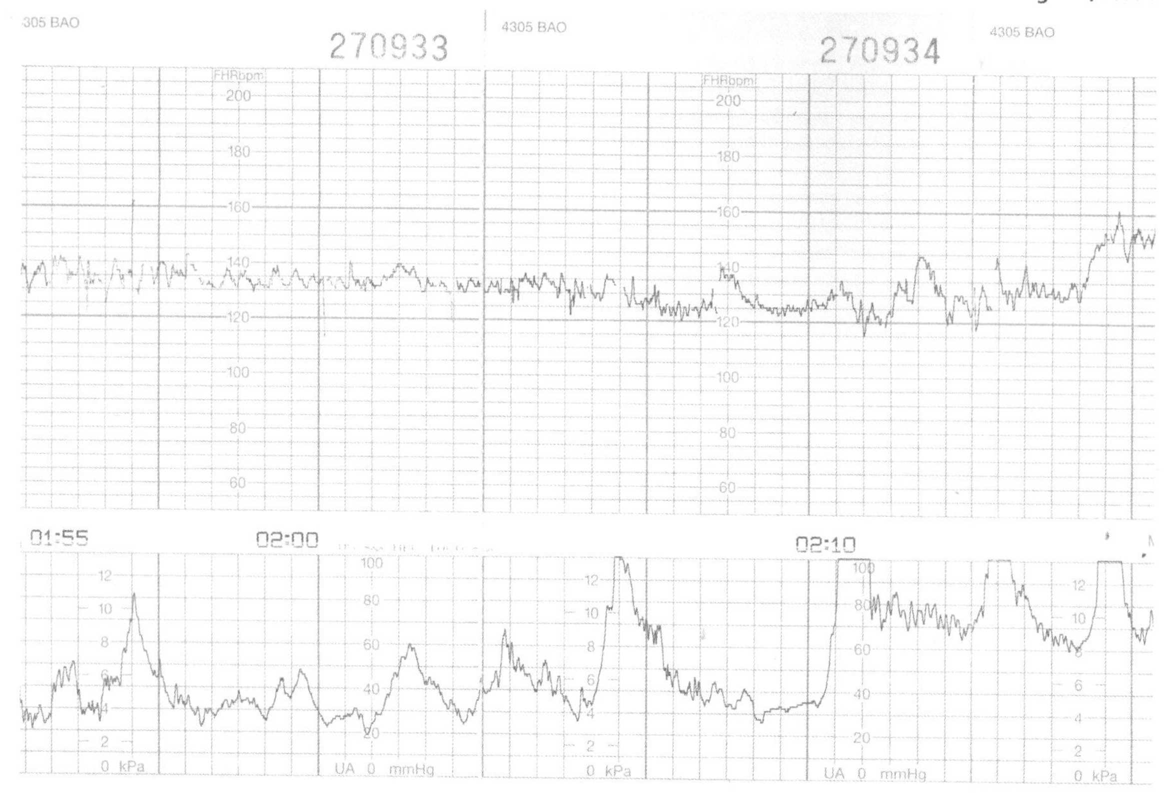

HISTORY

Gravida 3, para 2.

Past history

Previous caesarean section for breech presentation, normal birth since.
No medical disorders, no other problems noted.

Antenatal period

Planned vaginal birth.
Growth good, on 90th centile.
Admitted at 38 weeks in spontaneous labour at 01.30 hours.

Labour

01.45

Vaginal examination performed, cervical os 7 cm dilated, membranes intact.
External continuous electronic monitoring of the fetal heart commenced in view of previous caesarean section.

01.55

CTG (Fig. 4.4, Part 1).

CTG

1. What do you notice about the baseline?
2. What do you notice about the baseline variability?
3. What periodic changes, if any, are present?
4. What do you notice about the uterine activity?
5. Would you categorise this CTG as normal/suspicious/pathological?
6. What is the most probable cause of fetal heart rate abnormality shown on this trace?
7. What treatment and/or intervention would you consider necessary for this fetal heart rate pattern?

NOTES

1

2

3

4

5

6

7

ANALYSIS

1 Baseline 125–135 bpm — **Reassuring**
2 Variability 5–10 beats — **Reassuring**
3 No decelerations, accelerations present — **Reassuring**
4 Difficult to interpret but appear to be 3–4 in 10.
5 All features reassuring: CTG classified as normal.
6 No abnormalities present.
7 Attempts should be made to monitor the uterine activity more accurately.

Labour continued

02.35

Bulging membranes visible at intriotus. CTG remains normal as previously. No urges to push.

03.00

Spontaneous rupture of membranes, clear liquor, actively pushing.
CTG (Fig. 4.4, Part 2).

Case 4 continued over page.

Case 4 continued

Fig. 4.4, Part 2

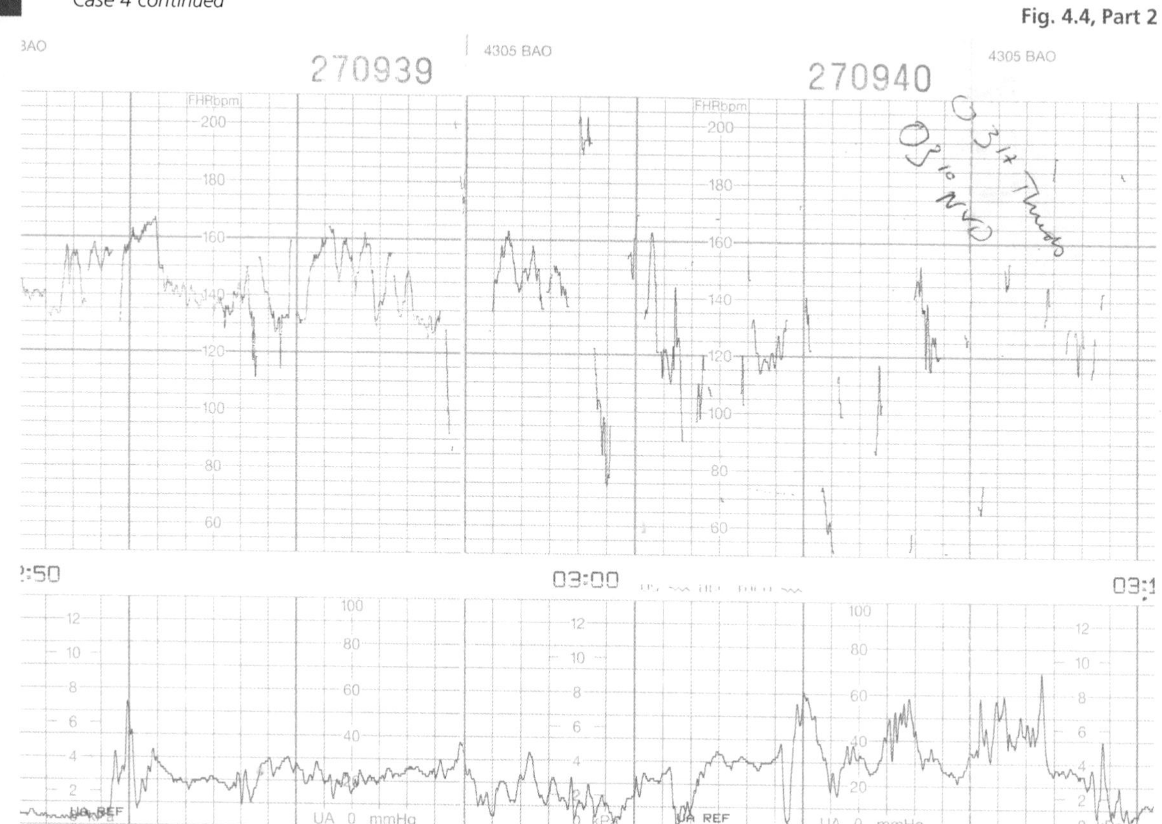

CTG

1 What do you notice about the baseline?
2 What do you notice about the baseline variability?
3 What periodic changes, if any, are present?
4 What do you notice about the uterine activity?
5 Would you categorise this CTG as normal/suspicious/pathological?
6 What is the most probable cause of fetal heart rate abnormality shown on this trace?
7 What treatment and/or intervention would you consider necessary for this fetal heart rate pattern?

NOTES

1

2

3

4

5

6

7

ANALYSIS

1	Baseline 130–135 bpm	**Reassuring**
2	Variability 5–10 beats	**Reassuring**
3	Accelerations present	**Reassuring**
	Atypical variable declerations for last 10 minutes	**Abnormal**

4 Contractions not monitored adequately.

5 One abnormal feature: the CTG is classified as pathological.

6 Variable decelerations are caused by cord compression. Atypical variables suggest a degree of hypoxia. This is a typical pattern of late second stage of labour.

7 In this case labour has progressed quickly and the fetus is descending through the birth canal. The CTG has been normal beforehand, which is reassuring. If good progress was not being made in the second stage of labour then consideration should be given to expediting birth.

OUTCOME

03.10

Normal birth, cord around the neck loosely.
Live boy, Apgar score 8/1 9/5.
Birthweight 3.800 kg.

Cord gases	pH	Base excess (mmol/l)
UA	6.99	16.1
UV	7.35	6.1

DISCUSSION

The arterial blood cord gases show a low pH and a high base excess. There is a large arteriovenous difference, suggestive of an acute acidaemia. The baby was behaving normally and did not display any concerning signs. This demonstrates the rapidity of the fall in fetal blood pH during the second stage even though the CTG has been normal previously.

Bradycardia

SECTION 2

Fig. 4.5

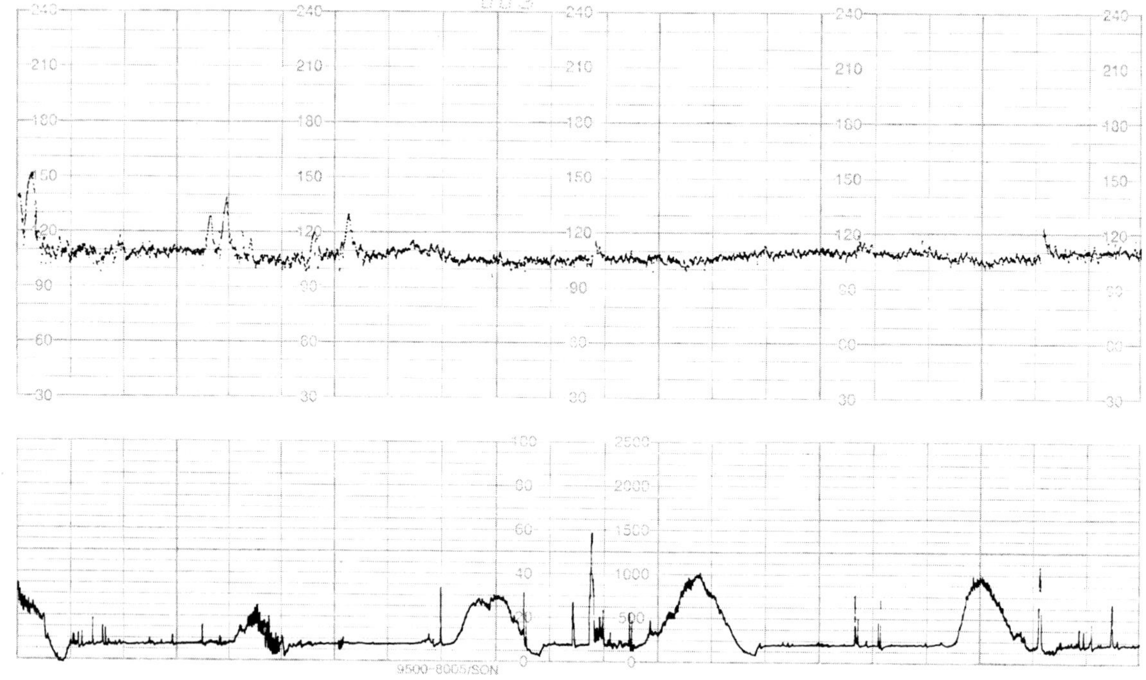

HISTORY

23-year-old gravida 1, para 0.

Past history

Nil relevant.

Antenatal period

Normal.
Admitted at 41 weeks with contractions.

Labour

07.00 hours

Cervical os 3 cm dilated.
Artificial rupture of membranes — clear liquor draining.
Fetal scalp electrode applied.
Contractions monitored externally.

08.15 hours

CTG (Fig. 4.5).

CTG

1 What do you notice about the baseline?
2 What do you notice about the baseline variability?
3 What periodic changes, if any, are present?
4 What do you notice about the uterine activity?
5 Would you categorise this CTG as normal/suspicious/pathological?
6 What is the most probable cause of fetal heart rate abnormality shown on this trace?
7 What treatment and/or intervention would you consider necessary for this fetal heart rate pattern?

NOTES

1

2

3

4

5

6

7

ANALYSIS

1 Baseline 100–110 bpm **Non-reassuring**
2 Variability 5 beats **Reassuring**
3 No decelerations, some accelerations **Reassuring**
4 Contracting 2 in 10 minutes, varying in strength.
5 One non-reassuring feature, baseline less than 110 bpm: CTG categorised as suspicious.
6 Low baseline, although some accelerations are occurring.
7 Although the baseline is low, there are reassuring features on the CTG; accelerations are a good sign of fetal well-being and are present. No drugs have been administered that may affect the fetal heart baseline. This is a low-risk pregnancy and the baby is well grown. It would therefore be acceptable to assume that there is no fetal compromise at the moment. The woman and her partner should be informed of the categorisation of the CTG and consent sought to continue the CTG.

OUTCOME

10.00 hours

Cervical os 5 cm dilated.
CTG unchanged.
Fetal blood sampling attempted – failed.
Decision made to deliver.
Caesarean section performed.
Live boy.
Apgar score 9/1 9/5, birthweight 3.650 kg.
No cord blood sample available for analysis.

DISCUSSION

The outcome in this case was good. Questions may arise as to why a fetal blood sample was deemed necessary at this point. The baseline remained low but other reassuring features were present: accelerations and normal variability. Whatever the reasons for the decision to perform the fetal blood sampling, when unable to obtain a sample the decision to proceed to caesarean section was correct. Generally, fetal blood sampling is recommended when a CTG is classified as pathological (NCCWCH 2007).

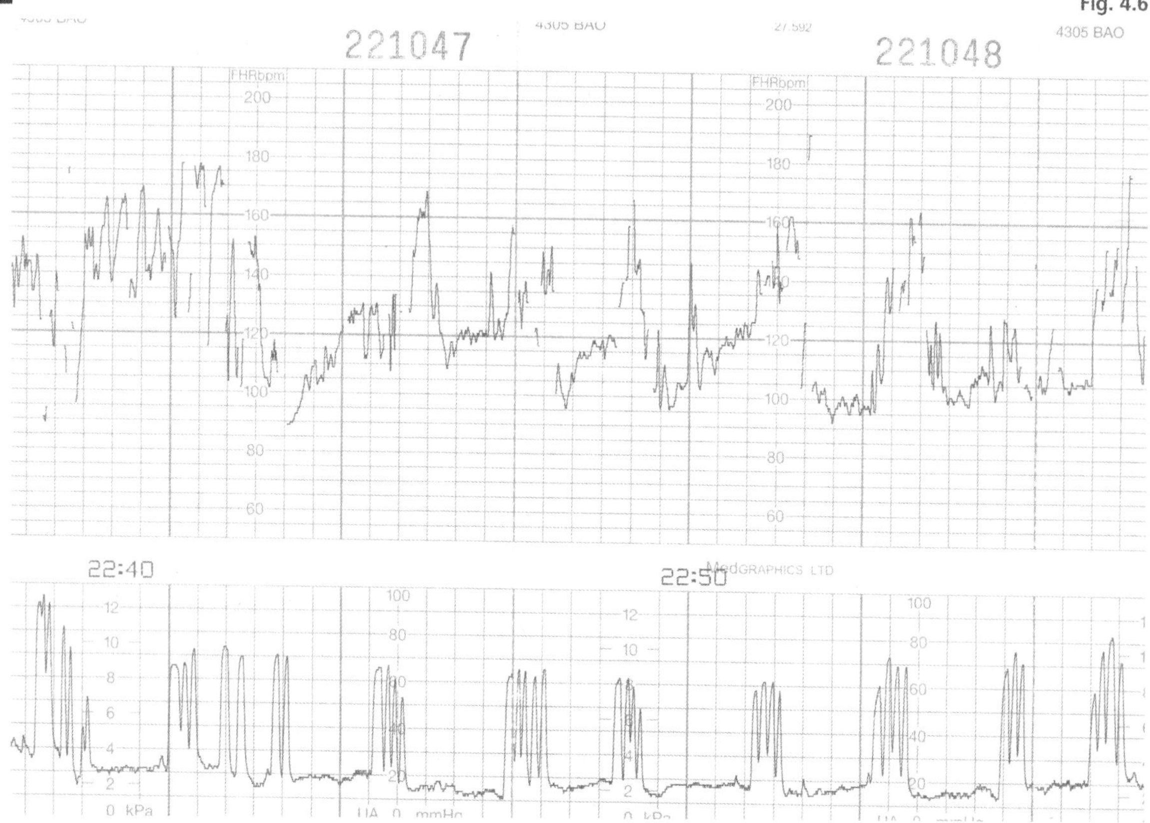

Fig. 4.6

HISTORY

19-year-old gravida 1, para 0.

Past history

No problems identified.

Antenatal period

Low risk, under midwife-led care.
Good growth, baby on 90th centile on symphysiofundal height measurement.
Admitted at 40 + 4 in spontaneous labour.

Labour

On admission in labour contractions were 4:10. The fetal heart was auscultated and the rate recorded as 105 bpm. This was rechecked and found to be the same. A CTG was commenced.
Vaginal examination revealed the cervix to be effaced and thin, the cervical os 6 cm dilated.
No analgesia was used.

Labour continued

Progress in labour was good: the CTG was normal with a low baseline.
Four hours after admission second stage of labour was diagnosed and active pushing commenced.
CTG (Fig. 4.6).

CTG

1. What do you notice about the baseline?
2. What do you notice about the baseline variability?
3. What periodic changes, if any, are present?
4. What do you notice about the uterine activity?
5. Would you categorise this CTG as normal/suspicious/pathological?
6. What is the most probable cause of fetal heart rate abnormality shown on this trace?
7. What treatment and/or intervention would you consider necessary for this fetal heart rate pattern?

NOTES

1

2

3

4

5

6

7

ANALYSIS

1 Baseline 100 bpm, although it is not easy to define. This could be a low baseline with accelerations or a higher baseline with decelerations. We do know that the baseline has been low throughout labour so it is reasonable to assume that the baseline remains low **Non-reassuring**
2 Variability 5–10 beats **Reassuring**
3 No decelerations, some accelerations: see comment on baseline **Reassuring**
4 Contracting 3–4 in 10 minutes, obvious signs of pushing.
5 One non-reassuring feature, baseline less than 110 bpm: CTG categorised as suspicious.
6 Low baseline, although some accelerations are occurring.
7 Although the baseline is low, there are reassuring features on the CTG: accelerations are a good sign of fetal well-being and are present. The baby is well grown and no problems have been identified during the antenatal period. Providing good progress is being made during the second stage of labour no intervention should be necessary.

OUTCOME

Normal birth occurred 10 minutes after the end of the CTG.
Baby boy, Apgar scores 9/1 9/5, birthweight 4.400 kg.
Cord blood analysis results fall into a normal range.

Cord gases	pH	Base excess (mmol/l)
UA	7.20	9
UV	7.29	8.5

Fig. 4.7

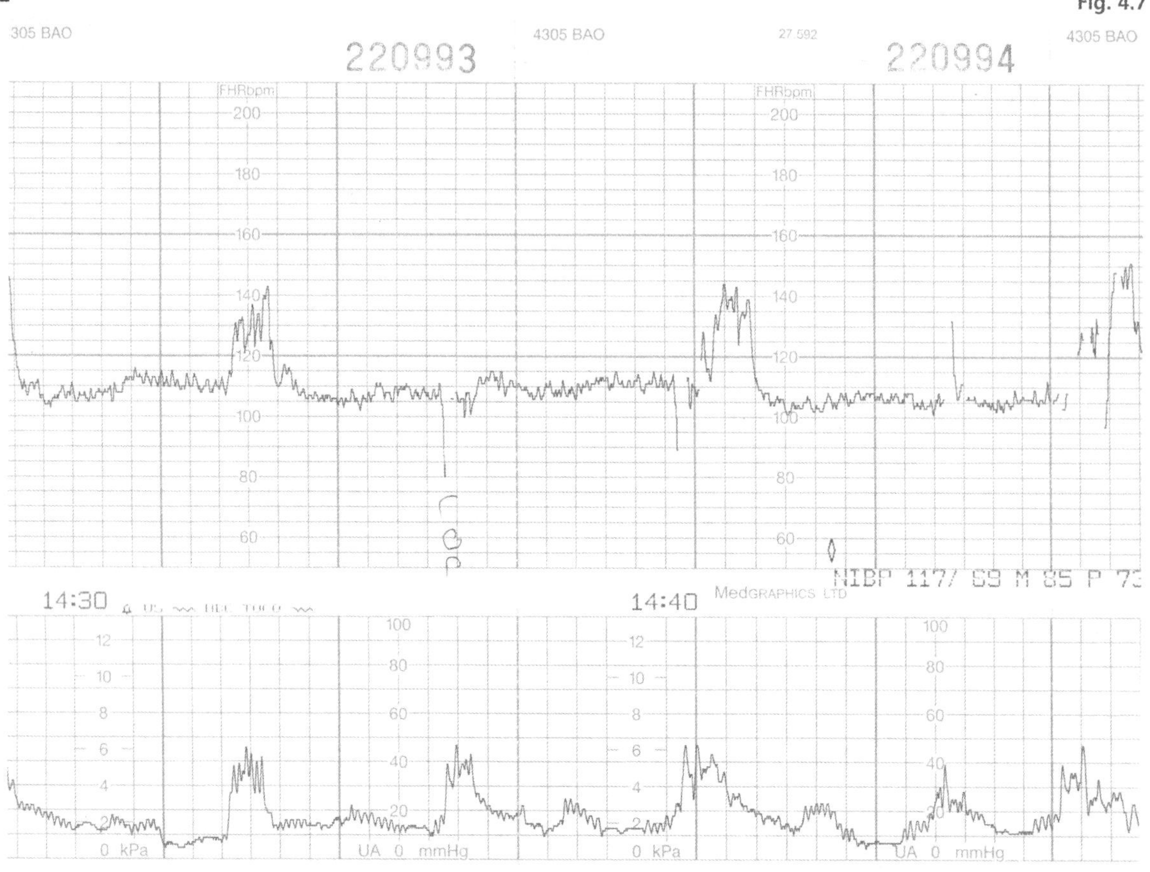

HISTORY

24-year-old gravida 2, para 0 + 1.

Past history

Asthmatic.

Antenatal period

No problems identified, low risk under midwife-led care. Admitted at 41 + 5 weeks in spontaneous labour.

Labour

On admission contractions 3:10. Fetal heart auscultated at 105 bpm. A CTG was commenced in view of this. CTG (Fig. 4.7).

CTG

1. What do you notice about the baseline?
2. What do you notice about the baseline variability?
3. What periodic changes, if any, are present?
4. What do you notice about the uterine activity?
5. Would you categorise this CTG as normal/suspicious/pathological?
6. What is the most probable cause of fetal heart rate abnormality shown on this trace?
7. What treatment and/or intervention would you consider necessary for this fetal heart rate pattern?

NOTES

1

2

3

4

5

6

7

ANALYSIS

1	Baseline 105 bpm	**Non-reassuring**
2	Variability 5 beats	**Reassuring**
3	No decelerations	**Reassuring**
	Accelerations present	**Reassuring**

4 Contracting 3 in 10 minutes.

5 One non-reassuring feature, baseline less than 110 bpm: CTG categorised as suspicious.

6 Low baseline, although accelerations are occurring.

7 Although the baseline is low, there are reassuring features on the CTG; accelerations are a good sign of fetal wellbeing and are present. The baby is well grown and no problems have been identified during the antenatal period. No intervention is necessary. If the woman prefers the fetal heart rate to be monitored by intermittent auscultation this should be possible with intermittent CTGs during labour.

OUTCOME

A vaginal examination was performed, the cervix effaced and thinning, the cervical os was 4 cm dilated, the membranes were ruptured artificially, clear liquor draining. Occipitoposterior position defined. CTG remained in progress.

The fetal heart baseline remained at 105 beats throughout labour.

Epidural analgesia was commenced and second stage of labour diagnosed 12 hours following CTG.

Birth was aided by vacuum extraction.

Live girl, Apgar score 9/1 9/5.

Birthweight 3.200 kg.

No cord blood samples available.

Tachycardia

SECTION 3

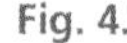
Fig. 4.8

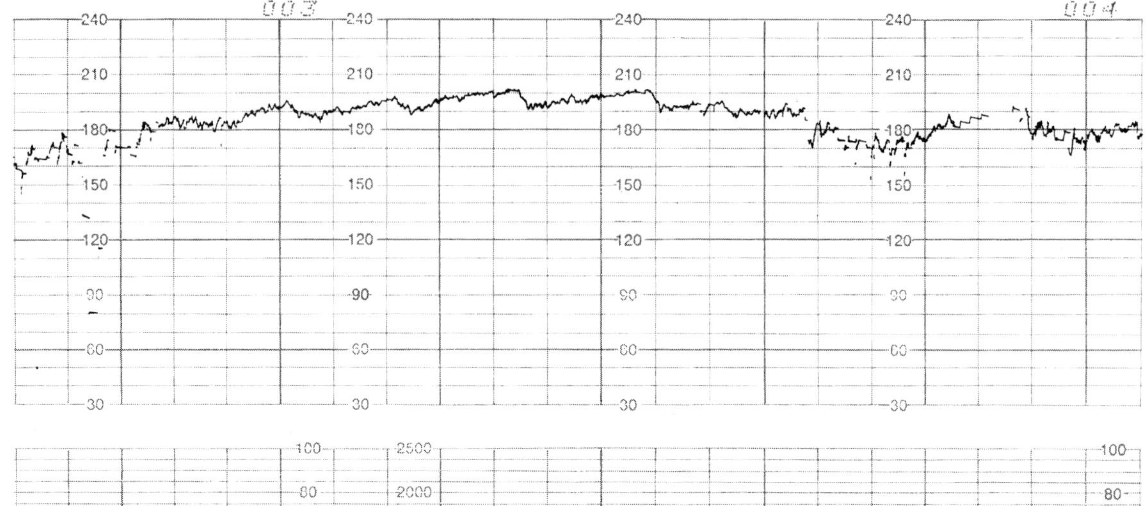

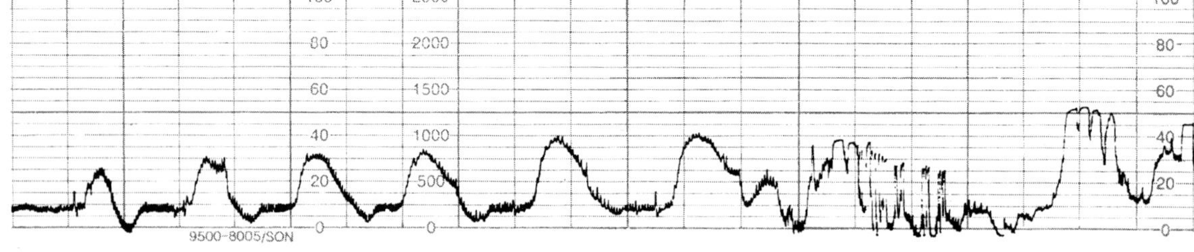

HISTORY

25-year-old gravida 1, para 0.

Past history

Nil relevant.

Antenatal period

Normal.
Admitted at 40 weeks, contracting 1 in 5 minutes for 2 hours.

Labour

19.30 hours

Cervical os 3 cm dilated.
Artificial rupture of membranes – clear liquor draining.
Fetal scalp electrode applied.
Contractions monitored externally.

22.30 hours

Cervical os 5 cm dilated.

22.45 hours

Epidural analgesia commenced.

02.30 hours

Cervical os 6 cm dilated.
CTG normal, baseline 140 bpm.

Labour continued

05.30 hours

Cervical os 8 cm dilated.

08.30 hours

Cervical os 9.5 cm dilated.
Clear liquor draining.
Maternal temperature 37.2 °C.

09.45 hours

Second stage of labour diagnosed.
CTG (Fig. 4.8).

CTG

1. What do you notice about the baseline?
2. What do you notice about the baseline variability?
3. What periodic changes, if any, are present?
4. What do you notice about the uterine activity?
5. Would you categorise this CTG as normal/suspicious/pathological?
6. What is the most probable cause of fetal heart rate abnormality shown on this trace?
7. What treatment and/or intervention would you consider necessary for this fetal heart rate pattern?

NOTES

1

2

3

4

5

6

7

ANALYSIS

1 Baseline 190–200 bpm — **Abnormal**
2 Variability less than 5 beats — **Non-reassuring**
3 No decelerations, no accelerations — **Reassuring**
4 Contracting 4 in 10 minutes, varying in strength.
5 There is one non-reassuring feature and one abnormal feature: the CTG is categorised as pathological.
6 The baseline fetal heart rate has increased during the labour. A mild maternal pyrexia was documented over 1 hour ago and may have increased. It is possible that the decrease in variability could be due to fetal sleep; however, because of the baseline tachycardia as well, fetal compromise should not be excluded.
7 Change maternal position. Reassess maternal temperature.
If pyrexia is evident, infection must be considered and appropriate treatment initiated.
Observe the colour of any liquor seen to exclude meconium staining and signs of infection.
The CTG is classified as pathological, therefore a fetal blood sample should be obtained.

OUTCOME

10.00 hours

Maternal temperature was not rechecked, fetal blood sample was not obtained.
Pushing was commenced.
CTG unchanged.

10.30 hours

No progress.
Straight forceps delivery.
Live girl.

Apgar score 7/1 9/5.
Birthweight 3.460 kg.
No cord gases were available for analysis.
No signs of infection were evident.

Fig. 4.9

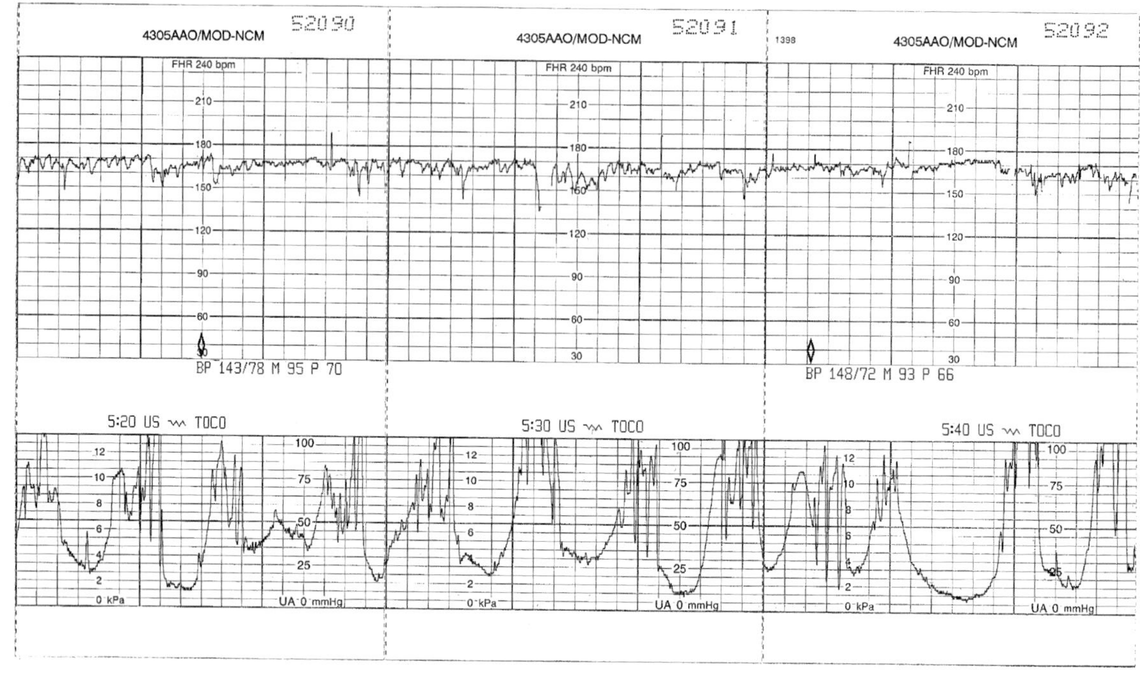

HISTORY

34-year-old gravida 3, para 0 + 2.

Past history

Two previous first-trimester abortions.
No significant medical or surgical history.
Antenatal period progressed normally, well-grown baby on serial symphysiofundal height measurements.
Admitted at 42 weeks' gestation for surgical induction of labour due to postdates pregnancy.

Labour

11.00 hours

Artificial rupture of membranes – clear liquor draining.
Syntocinon (oxytocin) infusion commenced.
Fetal heart and contractions monitored externally.

16.00 hours

Cervical os 4 cm dilated.
Clear liquor draining.
CTG normal, baseline 140 bpm.
Syntocinon infusion remains in progress.

CTG

1 What do you notice about the baseline?
2 What do you notice about the baseline variability?
3 What periodic changes, if any, are present?
4 What do you notice about the uterine activity?
5 Would you categorise this CTG as normal/suspicious/pathological?
6 What is the most probable cause of fetal heart rate abnormality shown on this trace?
7 What treatment and/or intervention would you consider necessary for this fetal heart rate pattern?

Labour continued

17.30 hours

Epidural analgesia commenced.

19.00 hours

Cervical os 8 cm dilated.
CTG normal.
Syntocinon infusion remains in progress.
Epidural effective.

21.00 hours

Second stage of labour diagnosed.
Maternal temperature 37.6 °C, pulse 100 bpm.
CTG (Fig. 4.9).

NOTES

1

2

3

4

5

6

7

ANALYSIS

1	Baseline 165–170 bpm	**Non-reassuring**
2	Variability 5–10 beats	**Reassuring**
3	No decelerations, no accelerations. The absence of accelerations is not considered to be a non-reassuring sign.	**Reassuring**

4 Contracting 3–4 in 10 minutes.
5 One non-reassuring feature present: the CTG is classified as suspicious.
6 The maternal temperature is raised so this is a potential cause of the tachycardia. Consideration should also be given to the possibility of dehydration in the woman.
7 Monitor mother's temperature and pulse, record on CTG in addition to labour record. Consider taking blood cultures and treat with antibiotics. Consider fluid replacement.

OUTCOME

21.30 hours

Commenced pushing.

22.15 hours

No progress being made, prepared for instrumental delivery.

22.40 hours

Straight forceps delivery.
Live boy.
Apgar score 5/1 9/5.
Birthweight 3.500 kg.
Cord gases: pH 7.33, base excess −10.7 mmol/l, within normal limits. However it is not certain if this was a venous or arterial sample; therefore acidaemia cannot be excluded. It is important that both vessels are sampled to obtain a result that can be accurately interpreted.
Baby's temperature 37.2 °C; ear, nose and cord swabs obtained, no growth.
No evidence of infection in the woman, temperature settled to normal within 2 hours of birth.

DISCUSSION

The degree of maternal fluid loss should not be underestimated during labour, particularly when it has been long, the woman has been vomiting or when it is particularly hot weather. Dehydration can lead to maternal tachycardia and subsequent fetal tachycardia. Women should be encouraged to maintain fluid balance during labour and accurate measurements of input and output completed.

Fig. 4.10

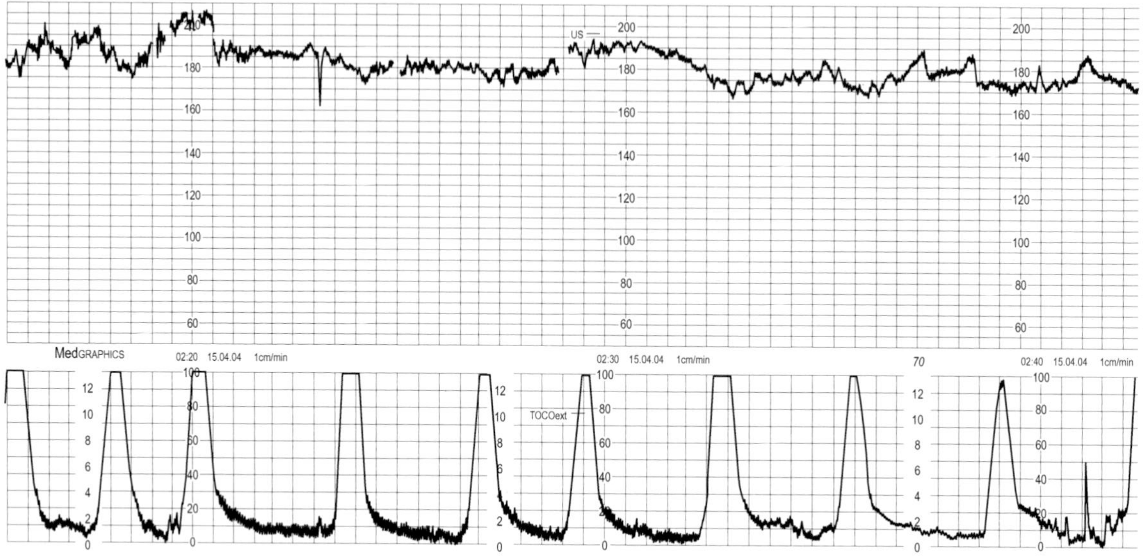

HISTORY

36-year-old gravida 2, para 1.

Past history

Previous normal delivery

Antenatal period

Normal.
Admitted at 40 weeks' gestation with contractions 1:5 for 3 hours.
Vaginal assessment revealed the cervix to be 1 cm long and posterior. The cervical os was 1 cm dilated.
CTG (Fig. 4.10).

CTG

1 What do you notice about the baseline?
2 What do you notice about the baseline variability?
3 What periodic changes, if any, are present?
4 What do you notice about the uterine activity?
5 Would you categorise the CTG as normal/suspicious/pathological?
6 What is the most probable cause of fetal heart rate abnormality shown on this trace?
7 What treatment and/or intervention would you consider necessary for this fetal heart rate pattern?

NOTES

1

2

3

4

5

6

7

ANALYSIS

1 Baseline 170–180 bpm **Non-reassuring**
2 Variability 5–10 beats **Reassuring**
3 No decelerations, accelerations present **Reassuring**
4 Contractions 1:3.
5 There is one non-reassuring feature: the CTG is classified as suspicious.
6 Maternal pyrexia is a possibility. Fetal compromise is also a possibility, although all other features are reassuring, making this unlikely. Fetal movements are not marked so reactivity to excessive fetal movements cannot be ruled out.
7 Assess maternal temperature and pulse rate. Assess fetal movements. Repeat CTG after 1 hour.

OUTCOME

Maternal temperature 38.7 °C, pulse rate 110 bpm.
Paracetamol prescribed regularly.
Blood cultures taken and intravenous antibiotics commenced.
Pyrexia subsided and fetal tachycardia resolved.
Prostin induction of labour was performed the following day.
Normal birth of a live boy occurred 42 hours after admission.
Apgar scores 9 and 9.
No evidence of infection or chorioamnionitis.
Birthweight 4.100 kg.
No cord blood samples available for analysis.

Fig. 4.11

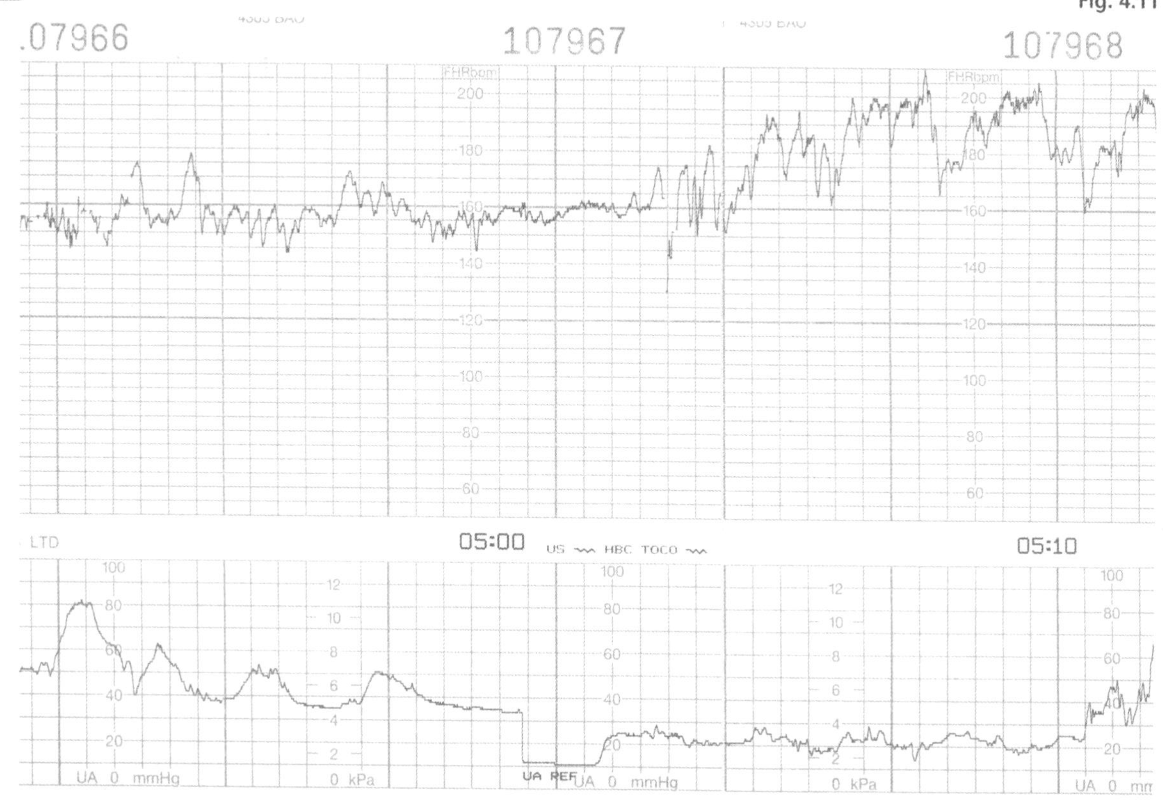

HISTORY

37-year-old gravida 1, para 0.

Past history

Normally fit and well, no problems identified.

Antenatal period

Developed raised blood pressure and proteinuria at 38 weeks' gestation, no medication required. Three days later complaining of generalised itching. Bile acids raised, therefore induction of labour advised.

Labour

Prostin induction of labour. Continuous CTG in progress as high-risk labour. CTG 2 hours after administration of second Prostin.
CTG (Fig. 4.11).

CTG

1 What do you notice about the baseline?
2 What do you notice about the baseline variability?
3 What periodic changes, if any, are present?
4 What do you notice about the uterine activity?
5 Would you categorise the CTG as normal/suspicious/pathological?
6 What is the most probable cause of fetal heart rate abnormality shown on this trace?
7 What treatment and/or intervention would you consider necessary for this fetal heart rate pattern?

NOTES

1

2

3

4

5

6

7

ANALYSIS

1 Baseline 160 bpm **Reassuring**
2 Variability 5–10 beats **Reassuring**
3 No decelerations, accelerations present **Reassuring**
4 Contractions irregular.
5 All features on CTG are currently reassuring: the CTG is classified as normal.
6 The baseline fetal heart rate is normal, although there is a rise in the second part of the CTG. It is important that fetal activity is assessed and documented on the CTG as this could be reactivity rather than a raise in baseline, which would be normal.
7 Document fetal activity.

OUTCOME

Artificial rupture of the membranes was performed 3 hours later, the cervix was 1 cm long and the os 2 cm dilated. Oxytocic infusion was commenced.
Labour progressed well: the CTG remained normal with a baseline of 160 bpm.
Normal birth 8 hours later.
Live girl, Apgar score 9/1 9/1. Birthweight 3.340 kg.

Reduced variability

SECTION 4

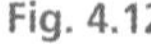
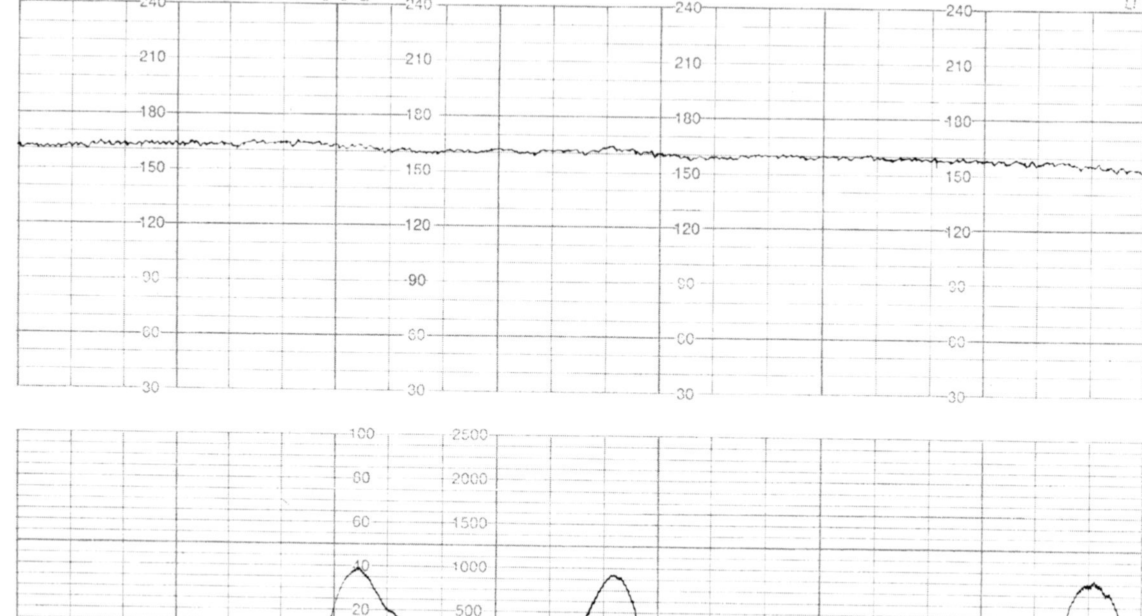
Fig. 4.12

HISTORY

25-year-old gravida 1, para 0.

Past history

Nil relevant.

Antenatal period

Normal.
Admitted at 40 weeks with contractions.

Labour

19.30 hours

Cervical os 3 cm dilated.
Artificial rupture of membranes – clear liquor draining.
Fetal scalp electrode applied.
Contractions monitored externally.
CTG normal.

20.20 hours

Pethidine 100 mg and Sparine 25 mg given intramuscularly.

20.40 hours

CTG (Fig. 4.12).

CTG

1 What do you notice about the baseline?
2 What do you notice about the baseline variability?
3 What periodic changes, if any, are present?
4 What do you notice about the uterine activity?
5 Would you categorise the CTG as normal/suspicious/pathological?
6 What is the most probable cause of fetal heart rate abnormality shown on this trace?
7 What treatment and/or intervention would you consider necessary for this fetal heart rate pattern?

NOTES

1

2

3

4

5

6

7

ANALYSIS

1 Baseline 160 bpm **Reassuring**
2 Variability little or none present **Non-reassuring**
3 No accelerations or decelerations **Reassuring**
4 Contractions irregular, 1–2 in 10 minutes.
5 There is one non-reassuring feature: the CTG is classified as suspicious.
6 In view of normal CTG prior to analgesia, possibly pethidine-induced.
7 Observe for further abnormalities. If pattern persists for longer than 90 minutes, the variability would become an abnormal feature, classifying the CRG as pathological and fetal blood sampling would be indicated.

OUTCOME

02.00 hours

Cervical os 6 cm dilated.
CTG now normal.

07.30 hours

Second stage of labour diagnosed.

08.20 hours

Normal birth.
Live girl.
Apgar score 7/1.9/5.
Birthweight 4.040 kg.

Fig. 4.13

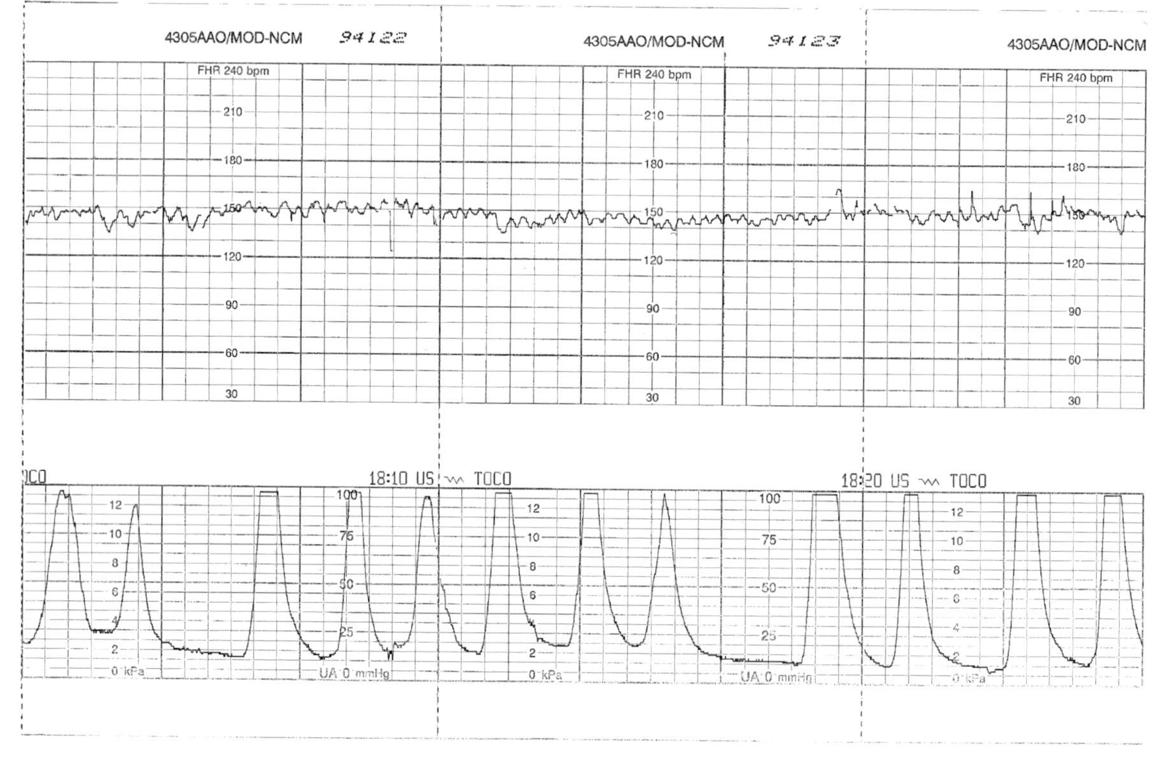

HISTORY

32-year-old gravida 4, para 2 + 1.

Past history

Previous mid-trimester abortion.

Antenatal period

Normal progress.
Admitted in spontaneous labour at 39 weeks' gestation.

Labour

17.00 hours

Cervical os 5 cm dilated, membranes intact.

17.58 hours

Pethidine 100 mg and Sparine 25 mg given intramuscularly.

18.00 hours

CTG (Fig. 4.13).

CTG

1. What do you notice about the baseline?
2. What do you notice about the baseline variability?
3. What periodic changes, if any, are present?
4. What do you notice about the uterine activity?
5. Would you categorise the CTG as normal/suspicious/pathological?
6. What is the most probable cause of fetal heart rate abnormality shown on this trace?
7. What treatment and/or intervention would you consider necessary for this fetal heart rate pattern?

NOTES

1

2

3

4

5

6

7

ANALYSIS

1 Baseline 145–150 bpm **Reassuring**
2 Variability – ? sinusoidal pattern initially, shows signs of reverting to normal variability towards end of portion of CTG. **Non-reassuring**
3 No decelerations
possibly small accelerations present just before 18.20 hours **Reassuring**
4 Contracting 4 in 10 minutes.
5 There is one non-reassuring feature: the CTG is classified as suspicious.
6 In view of normal variability previously, return to normal at end of CTG and absence of other abnormalities, probably pethidine-induced.
7 Continue to monitor the fetal heart. If pattern persists, consider artificial rupture of the membranes to assess the colour of the liquor with the woman's consent.

OUTCOME

Progressed rapidly to normal birth at 19.00 hours.
Live boy.
Apgar score 9/1 9/5.
Birthweight 2.960 kg.
No cord gases available.

Fig. 4.14

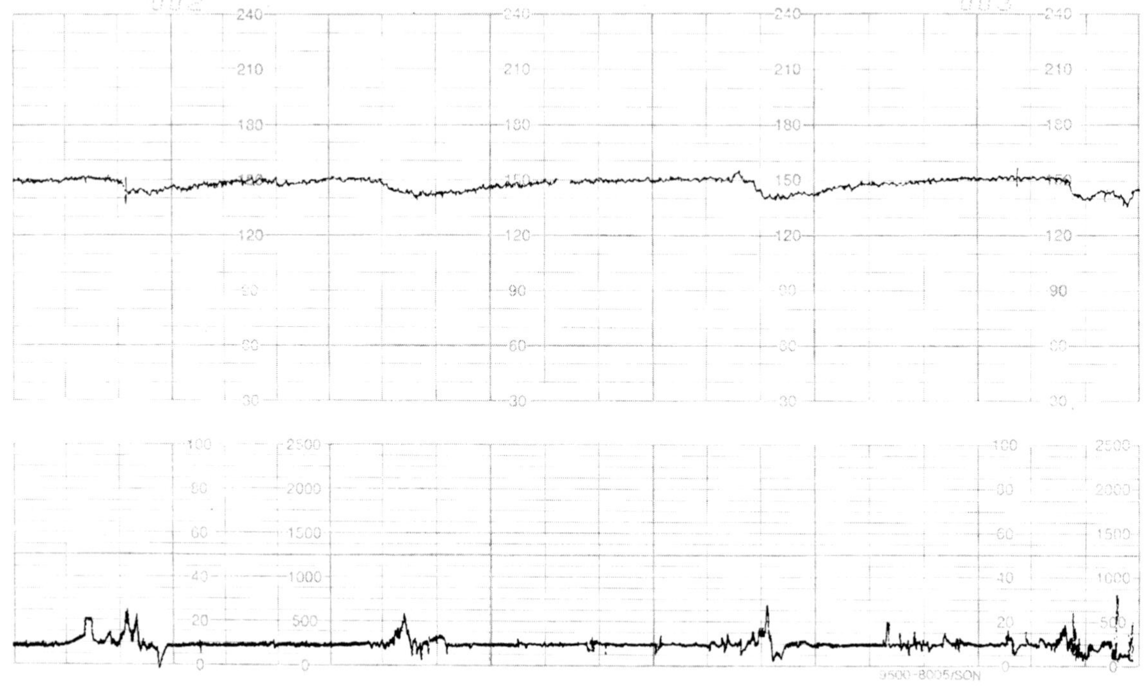

HISTORY

25-year-old gravida 2, para 0 + 1.

Past history

Deep venous thrombosis 4 years ago.

Antenatal history

Treated with prophylactic subcutaneous heparin from 16 weeks.
Well-grown baby on 50th centile on regular symphysiofundal height measurements.
Admitted at 40 weeks, contracting 1 in 5 minutes.

Labour

16.45 hours

Cervical os 2–3 cm dilated.
Artificial rupture of membranes – fresh, thick meconium-stained liquor draining.
Fetal scalp electrode applied.
Contractions monitored externally.
CTG (Fig. 4.14).

CTG

1. What do you notice about the baseline?
2. What do you notice about the baseline variability?
3. What periodic changes, if any, are present?
4. What do you notice about the uterine activity?
5. Would you categorise the CTG as normal/suspicious/pathological?
6. What is the most probable cause of fetal heart rate abnormality shown on this trace?
7. What treatment and/or intervention would you consider necessary for this fetal heart rate pattern?

NOTES

1

2

3

4

5

6

7

ANALYSIS

1 Baseline 145–150 bpm **Reassuring**
2 Variability little or absent **Non-reassuring**
3 Shallow decelerations, cannot be classified as contractions not monitored adequately
No evidence of accelerations. **Abnormal**
4 Contractions not monitored adequately.
5 There is one abnormal and one non-reassuring feature: the CTG is classified as pathological.
6 Decreased-variability decelerations, which look as though they may be late. If the transducer has detected some uterine pressure changes and the presence of fresh meconium must alert the professional to the real possibility of fetal compromise.
No drugs have been administered and we have no information about the fetal movements.
7 Ascertain the presence of normal fetal movements. Obtain a fetal blood sample if possible. Consider the need for immediate delivery.

OUTCOME

17.30 hours

Caesarean section performed.
Live boy.
Apgar score 8/1 10/5.
Birthweight 3.100 kg.
No cord bloods were available for analysis, although the Apgar scores were normal; a degree of hypoxia cannot be excluded.

Fig. 4.15

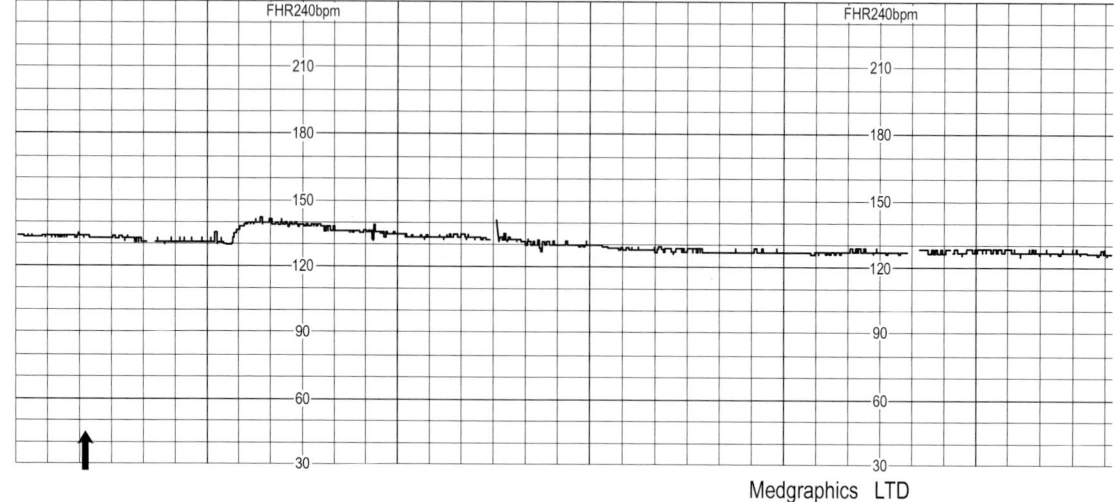

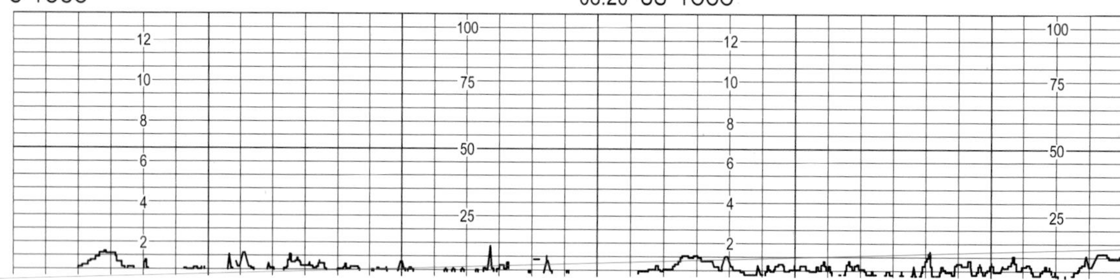

HISTORY

26-year-old gravida 2, para 1.

Past history

Previous forceps delivery for delay in second stage of labour.
No medical problems.

Antenatal period

Normal. Admitted at 37 weeks' gestation with a history of diminished fetal movements over the past 2 days.
No signs of labour.
CTG (Fig. 4.15).

CTG

1 What do you notice about the baseline?
2 What do you notice about the baseline variability?
3 What periodic changes, if any, are present?
4 What do you notice about the uterine activity?
5 Would you categorise the CTG as normal/suspicious/pathological?
6 What is the most probable cause of fetal heart rate abnormality shown on this trace?
7 What treatment and/or intervention would you consider necessary for this fetal heart rate pattern?

NOTES

1

2

3

4

5

6

7

ANALYSIS

1 Baseline 130 bpm — **Reassuring**
2 Variability absent — **Non-reassuring**
3 No decelerations, no accelerations — **Reassuring**
4 No contractions.
5 There is one non-reassuring feature: the CTG is classified as suspicious.
6 The reduced variability could be due to fetal sleep, or sedative drugs. The woman should be asked about any alcohol or drug consumption. However in view of the absent variability and history of altered fetal movements, fetal hypoxia must be considered.
7 Continue CTG. If the variability does not improve and continues for 90 minutes, this becomes an abnormal feature and the CTG classification changes to pathological.

OUTCOME

Maternal observations of blood pressure, pulse and temperature were normal. Vaginal assessment revealed the cervix to be 0.5 cm long, softening and posterior. The cervical os was 2 cm dilated. There was sufficient concern regarding the CTG in this instance that immediate delivery by caesarean section was performed.

A live girl was delivered with an Apgar score of 1/1 2/9.

Cord gases	pH	Base excess (mmol/l)
UA	7.28	6.6
UV	7.31	2.3

The cord blood sample results are within normal limits.

Birthweight 2.760 kg.

This baby sadly died at 3 hours of age. Consent was refused for postmortem examination.

DISCUSSION

The portion of CTG that is shown falls into a suspicious category; however other factors must be taken into account. Labour has not commenced and the woman has concerns that the baby has not been moving normally for 2 days. It is not necessary to wait until a CTG has become pathological to proceed with fetal blood sampling or delivery. The clinical picture must always be taken into account.

Fig. 4.16

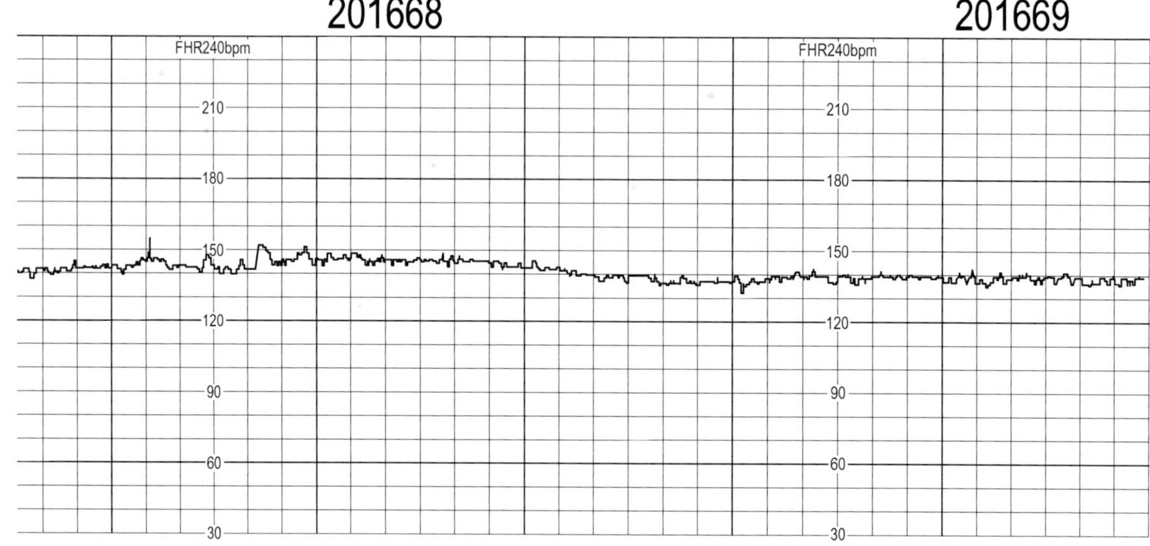

REF UA REF 18:00 US TOCO 18:10 US

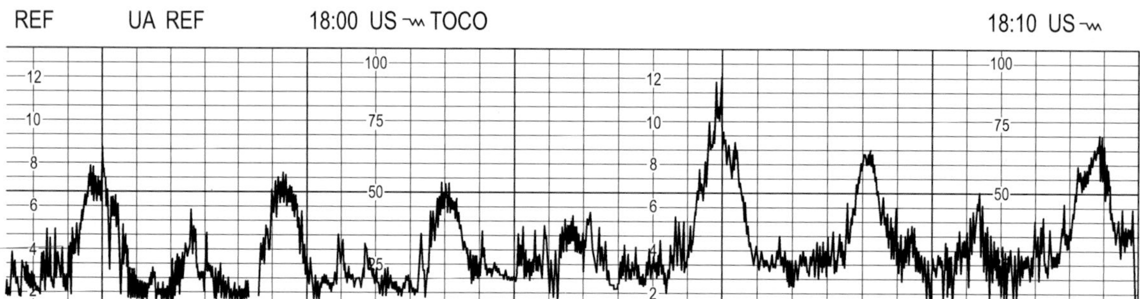

HISTORY

19-year-old gravida 1, para 0.

Past history

Nil of note.

Antenatal period

Three admissions in mid-trimester with low abdominal pain; no cause was found.
Admitted at 40 + 3 with contractions.
Vaginal assessment revealed the cervix to be effaced, thin and the os 4 cm dilated. The woman was transferred to the delivery suite.

Labour

Analgesia was requested and pethidine 100 mg was given. 35 minutes later CTG: fetal heart rate monitored by external transducer.
CTG (Fig. 4.16).

CTG

1. What do you notice about the baseline?
2. What do you notice about the baseline variability?
3. What periodic changes, if any, are present?
4. What do you notice about the uterine activity?
5. Would you categorise the CTG as normal/suspicious/pathological?
6. What is the most probable cause of fetal heart rate abnormality shown on this trace?
7. What treatment and/or intervention would you consider necessary for this fetal heart rate pattern?

NOTES

1

2

3

4

5

6

7

ANALYSIS

1 Baseline 140 bpm **Reassuring**
2 Variability less than 5 beats **Non-reassuring**
3 No decelerations, no accelerations **Reassuring**
4 Contractions not monitored adequately.
5 There is one non-reassuring feature: the CTG is classified as suspicious.
6 The most likely cause of the loss of fetal heart rate variability is the administration of pethidine. Fetal compromise should be considered if pattern continues beyond 90 minutes and the CTG would then move into a pathological classification.
7 Continue to observe CTG until parameters return to normal, then discontinue. As this woman was deemed low-risk for labour the reason why a CTG was commenced should be questioned. The administration of pethidine should not be a reason for a CTG as this may lead to other interventions when a decrease in variability inevitably occurs. The woman should be offered intermittent auscultation as the preferred method of fetal heart rate monitoring. If she chooses to have continuous monitoring the risks and benefits as explained to the woman must be documented in the case notes and her informed consent gained.

OUTCOME

Progressed well in labour.
Variability returned to normal after 60 minutes.
The CTG was discontinued and intermittent auscultation was used for the remainder of the labour.
A live boy was delivered 6 hours following the CTG.
Apgar score 9 and 9.
Birthweight 3.240 kg.

Fig. 4.17

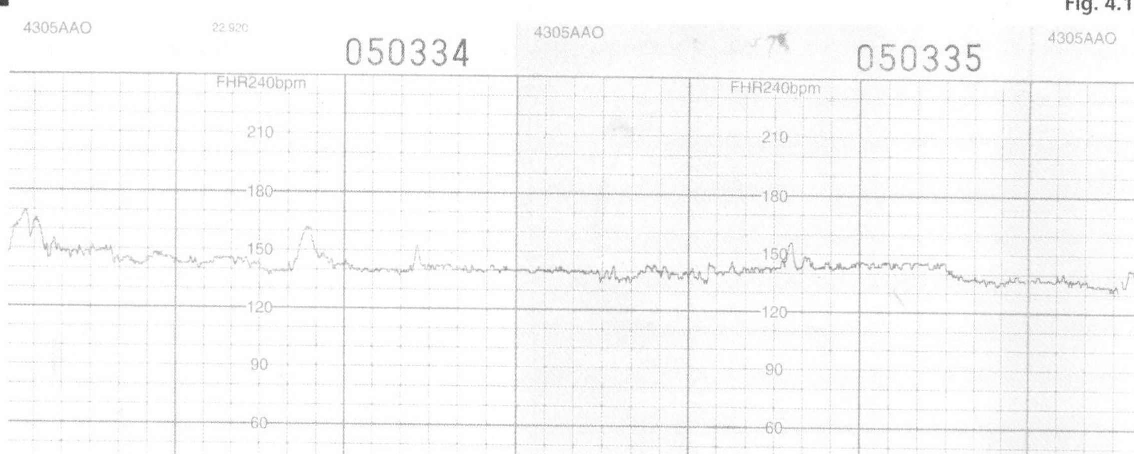

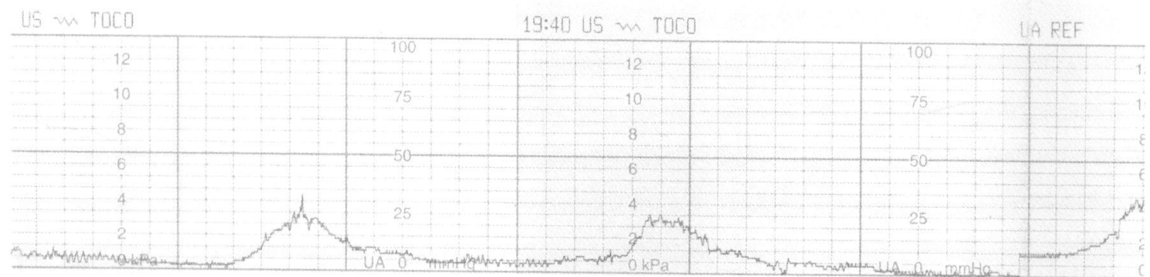

HISTORY

24-year-old gravida 1, para 0.

Past history

Normally fit and well.

Antenatal period

Normal progress.
Admitted in spontaneous labour at 40 + 4 weeks' gestation. Low risk.

Labour

Vaginal examination performed on admission; cervix, effaced and thinning, os 4–5 cm dilated. Mobilising, intermittent ausculatation as method of fetal heart rate monitoring.

3 hours later cervical dilatation unchanged. Membranes ruptured artificially, Oxytocic infusion commenced and continuous CTG commenced. CTG normal.

7 hours later, cervical os 9 cm dilated, Syntocinon infusion at 8 ml per hour.
CTG (Fig. 4.17).

CTG

1 What do you notice about the baseline?
2 What do you notice about the baseline variability?
3 What periodic changes, if any, are present?
4 What do you notice about the uterine activity?
5 Would you categorise the CTG as normal/suspicious/pathological?
6 What is the most probable cause of fetal heart rate abnormality shown on this trace?
7 What treatment and/or intervention would you consider necessary for this fetal heart rate pattern?

NOTES

1

2

3

4

5

6

7

ANALYSIS

1 Baseline 140 bpm **Reassuring**
2 Variability less than 5 beats. **Non-reassuring**
3 No decelerations **Reassuring**
Small accelerations present **Reassuring**
4 Contracting 2 in 10 minutes.
5 There is one non-reassuring feature: the CTG is classified as suspicious.
6 In view of normal variability previously, and no other abnormalities present, this could be a fetal sleep pattern and should return to normal variability within 90 minutes.
7 Continue to monitor the fetal heart.

OUTCOME

4 hours later caesarean section was performed for secondary arrest in labour.
Baby boy. Apgar score 8/1 9/5. Birthweight 3.330 kg.
Cord blood analysis: results within normal limits.

Cord gases	pH	Base excess (mmol/l)
UA	7.31	3.8
UV	7.32	2.6

Fig. 4.18, Part 1

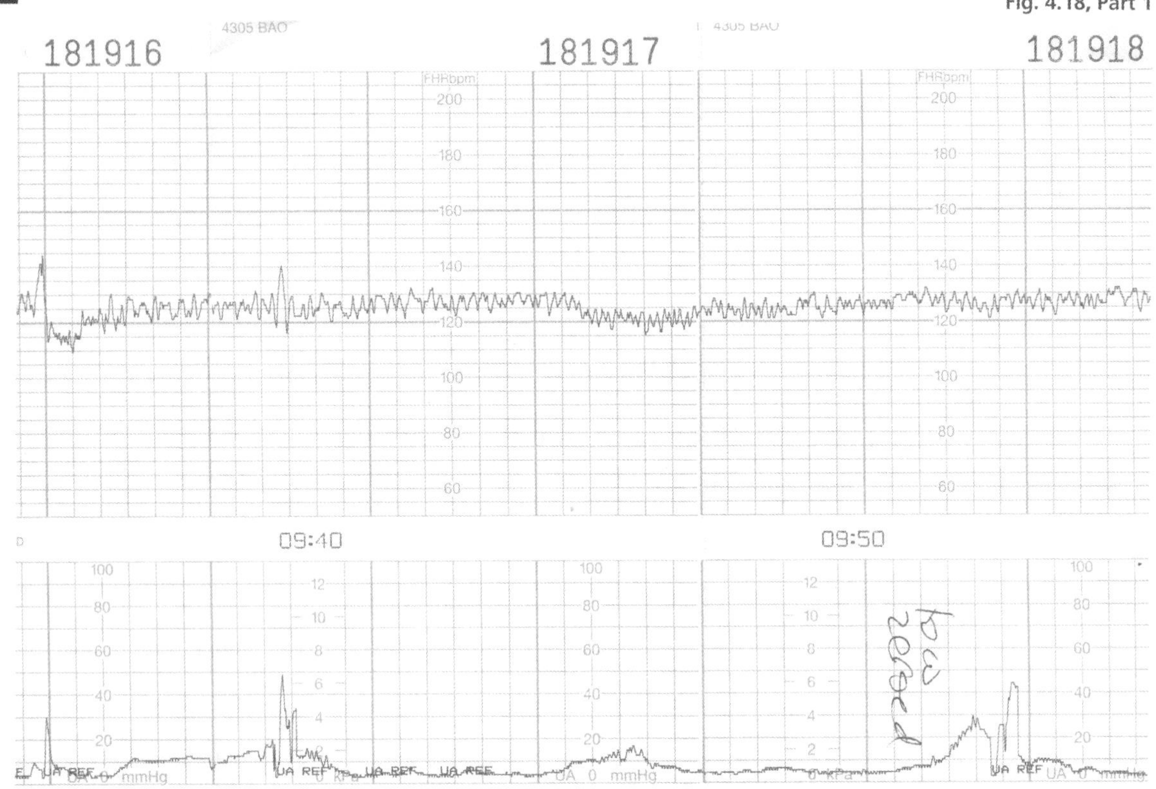

HISTORY

26-year-old gravida 1, para 0.

Past history

Nil of note, normally fit and well.

Antenatal period

No problems identified. Well-grown baby on 50th centile, regular symphysiofundal height measurements. Low risk, midwife-led care.

Admitted at 39 weeks with reduced fetal movements. CTG normal, normal Dopplers and liquor volume on scan. Two days later admitted in spontaneous labour. Fetal movements normal.

Labour

CTG was commenced.
CTG (Fig. 4.18, Part 1).

CTG

1 What do you notice about the baseline?
2 What do you notice about the baseline variability?
3 What periodic changes, if any, are present?
4 What do you notice about the uterine activity?
5 Would you categorise the CTG as normal/suspicious/pathological?
6 What is the most probable cause of fetal heart rate abnormality shown on this trace?
7 What treatment and/or intervention would you consider necessary for this fetal heart rate pattern?

NOTES

1

2

3

4

5

6

7

ANALYSIS

1 Baseline 125 bpm **Reassuring**
2 Variability less than 5 beats, sinusoidal-type pattern **Abnormal**
3 No decelerations, no accelerations **Reassuring**
4 Contractions not monitored adequately.
5 There is one abnormal feature: the CTG is classified as pathological.
6 The cause may be idiopathic. There is a history of reduced fetal movements, although they are normal at present. Fetal compromise should not be excluded as a cause.
7 The CTG should be continued and consideration given to performing a fetal blood sample as the CTG is pathological. As this woman was deemed low risk for labour the reason why a CTG was commenced should be questioned.

OUTCOME

Vaginal examination was performed, the cervix was thin and the os 3 cm dilated. Artificial rupture of the membranes was performed, clear liquor draining. 10 minutes later CTG reviewed.

Case 18 continued over page.

Case 18 continued

Fig. 4.18, Part 2

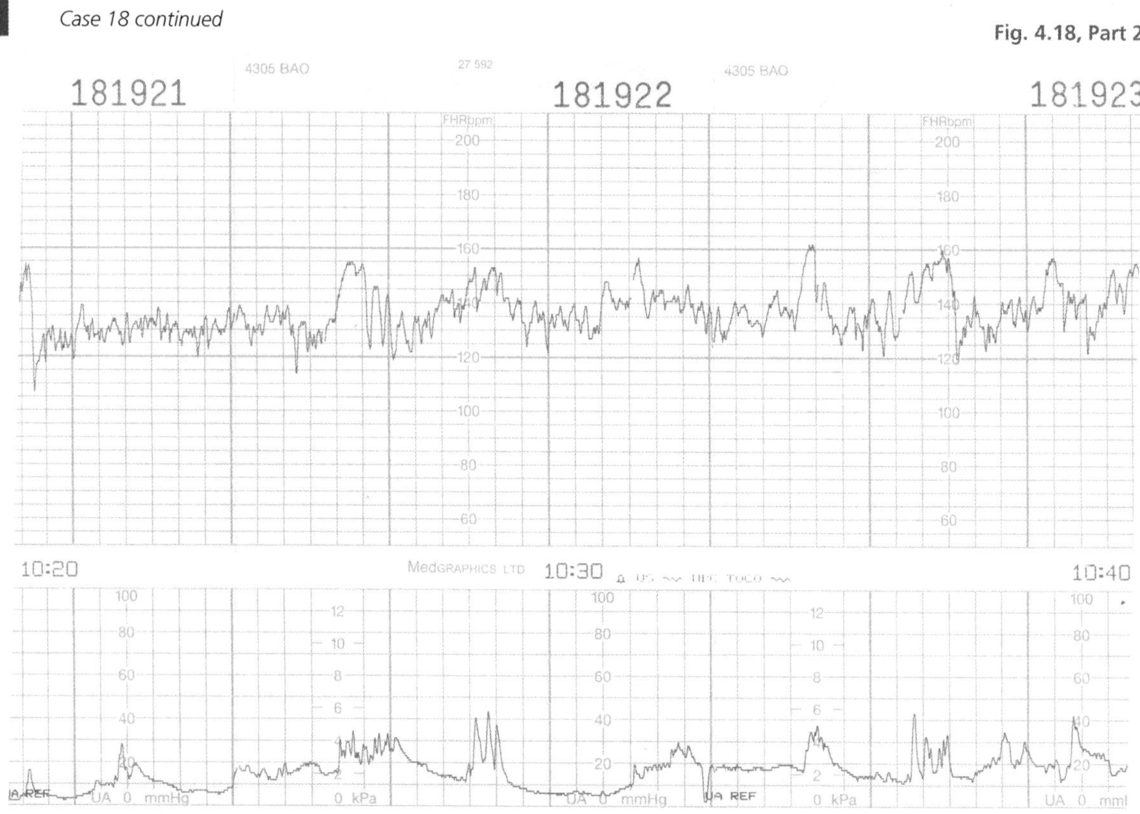

CTG (Fig. 4.18, Part 2)

1. Baseline 125 bpm **Reassuring**
2. Variability 5–10 beats **Reassuring**
3. No decelerations, accelerations present **Reassuring**
4. Contractions not monitored adequately.
5. All features are now reassuring: CTG is classified as normal.
6. As this is a low-risk labour, the CTG should be discontinued and intermittent auscultation recommended for fetal heart rate monitoring.

OUTCOME

Labour progressed well, although the CTG remained in progress. There is documentation in the labour record stating the reason for this is to ensure sinusoidal pattern does not return. This demonstrates a lack of confidence or knowledge in CTG interpretation. Fetal compromise will not be the cause of this pattern if it reverts to normal and no other features give cause for concern.

Normal birth 8 hours later.

Baby boy. Apgar score 9/1 9/5. Birthweight 3.560 kg.

Early decelerations

SECTION 5

Fig. 4.19

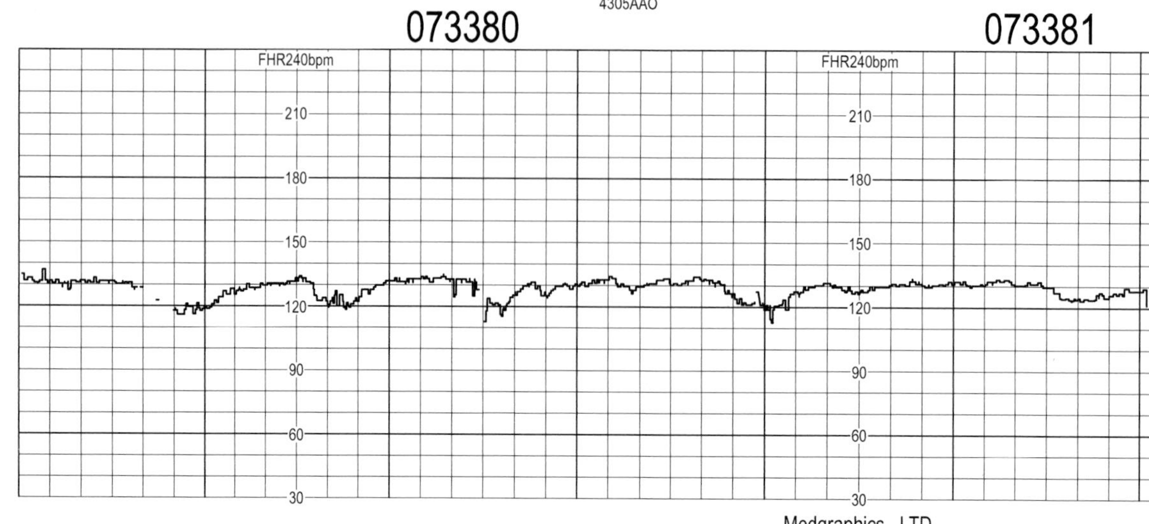

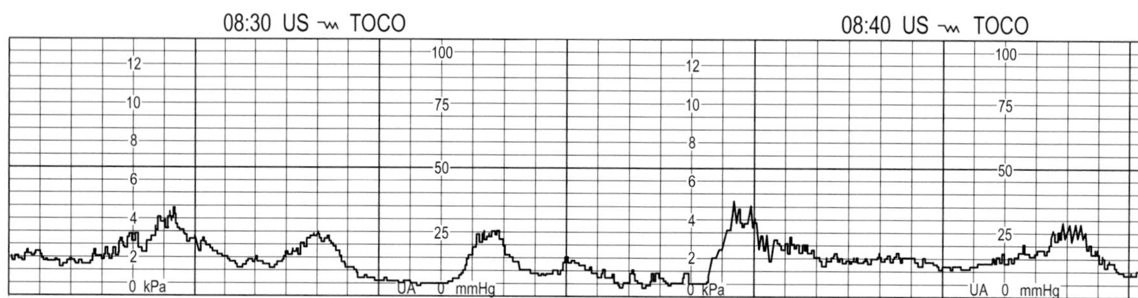

HISTORY

27-year-old gravida 3, para 2.

Past history

Nil relevant.

Antenatal period

Developed mild hypertension in last few weeks of pregnancy. No proteinuria, blood profile normal.

Admitted at 41 weeks' gestation in spontaneous labour.

Vaginal assessment revealed the cervix to be thin, well applied to presenting part and the cervical os 6 cm dilated.

Labour

Continuous fetal heart rate monitoring was initiated because of the hypertension. The cervical os is now 8 cm dilated.
CTG (Fig. 4.19).

CTG

1. What do you notice about the baseline?
2. What do you notice about the baseline variability?
3. What periodic changes, if any, are present?
4. What do you notice about the uterine activity?
5. Would you categorise the CTG as normal/suspicious/pathological
6. What is the most probable cause of fetal heart rate abnormality shown on this trace?
7. What treatment and/or intervention would you consider necessary for this fetal heart rate pattern?

NOTES

1

2

3

4

5

6

7

ANALYSIS

1 Baseline 130 bpm — **Reassuring**
2 Variability less than 5 beats — **Non-reassuring**
3 Early decelerations — **Reassuring**
4 Contractions 2–3:10
5 There is one non-reassuring feature: the CTG is classified as suspicious.
6 Head compression causing early decelerations. Decreased variability could be due to fetal sleep; if pattern persists beyond 90 minutes, fetal hypoxia should be considered.
7 Continue CTG in view of reduced variability. If this does not improve within 90 minutes this becomes an abnormal feature and the CTG classification changes to pathological.
Change maternal position to relieve head compression.
True early decelerations are not usually associated with fetal compromise.

OUTCOME

Variability returned to normal 15 minutes later, with accelerations also present.
Labour progresses well and a live girl was born with an Apgar score of 9/1 9/5.
Birthweight 3.900 kg.
Cord blood analysis results within normal limits.

Cord gases	pH	Base excess (mmol/l)
UA	7.23	4.2
UV	7.35	3.7

Fig. 4.20

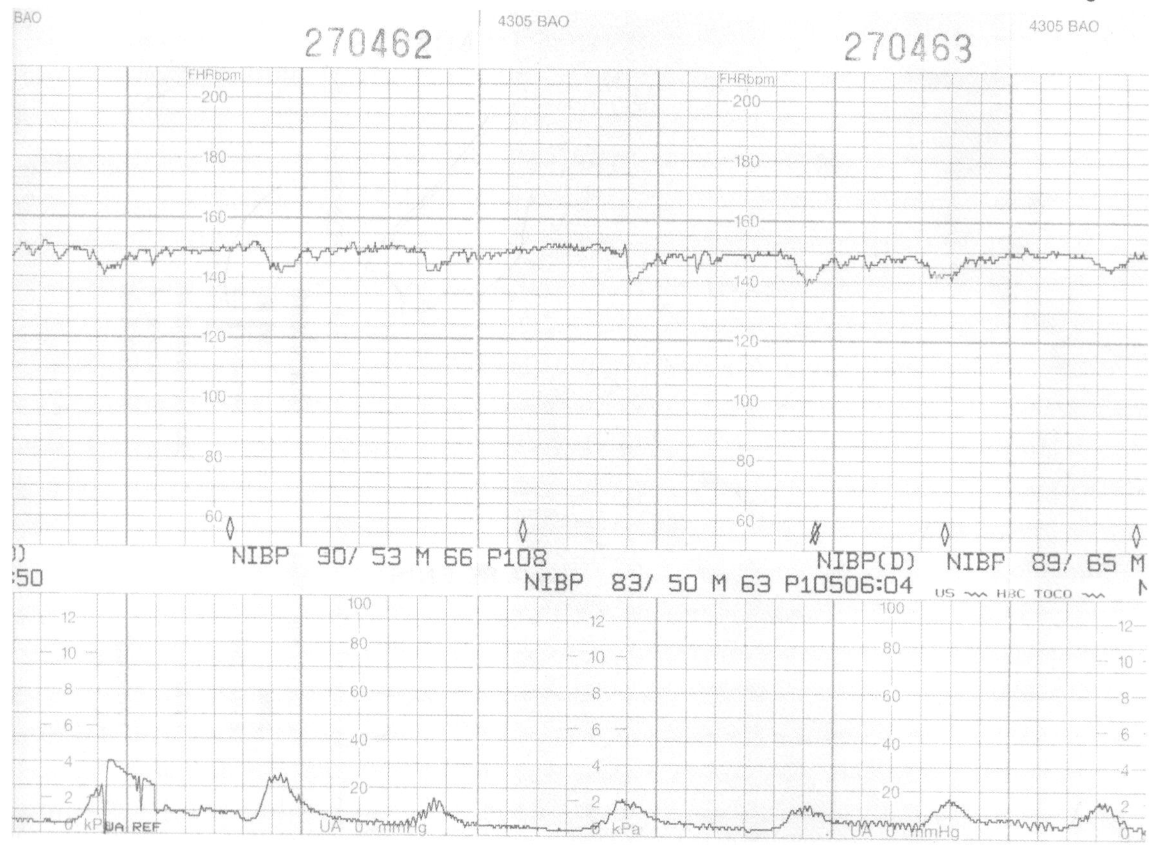

HISTORY

31-year-old gravida 1, para 0.

Past history

Body mass index 42.
Normally well.

Antenatal period

Normal glucose tolerance test at 28 weeks. Growth on 50th centile on regular symphysiofundal height measurements.

No problems identified.

40 + 5, membrane sweep performed.

Labour

40 + 10, Prostin induction of labour.

Artificial rupture of membranes performed 24 hours later. Clear liquor draining, cervix thinning, cervical os 4 cm dilated. Fetal heart monitored continuously with external transducer.
CTG (Fig. 4.20).

CTG

1 What do you notice about the baseline?
2 What do you notice about the baseline variability?
3 What periodic changes, if any, are present?
4 What do you notice about the uterine activity?
5 Would you categorise the CTG as normal/suspicious/pathological?
6 What is the most probable cause of fetal heart rate abnormality shown on this trace?
7 What treatment and/or intervention would you consider necessary for this fetal heart rate pattern?

NOTES

1

2

3

4

5

6

7

ANALYSIS

1 Baseline 150 bpm **Reassuring**
2 Variability 5 beats in places, although reduced in later part of CTG **Reassuring**
3 Early decelerations **Reassuring**
No accelerations
4 Contractions 3:10.
5 All features are reassuring: the CTG is classified as normal. Early decelerations do not cause fetal compromise.
6 Head compression causing early decelerations.
7 Continue CTG in view of decreased variability. Encourage woman to be mobile or move to left lateral to ease head compression.

OUTCOME

Oxytocic infusion commenced 4 hours later, no increase in cervical dilatation. CTG, early decelerations improved. Epidural anaesthesia commenced. Progressed to normal birth.

Live boy, Apgar score 9/1 9/5. Birthweight 3.780 kg.

Cord blood sample not obtained.

Fig. 4.21

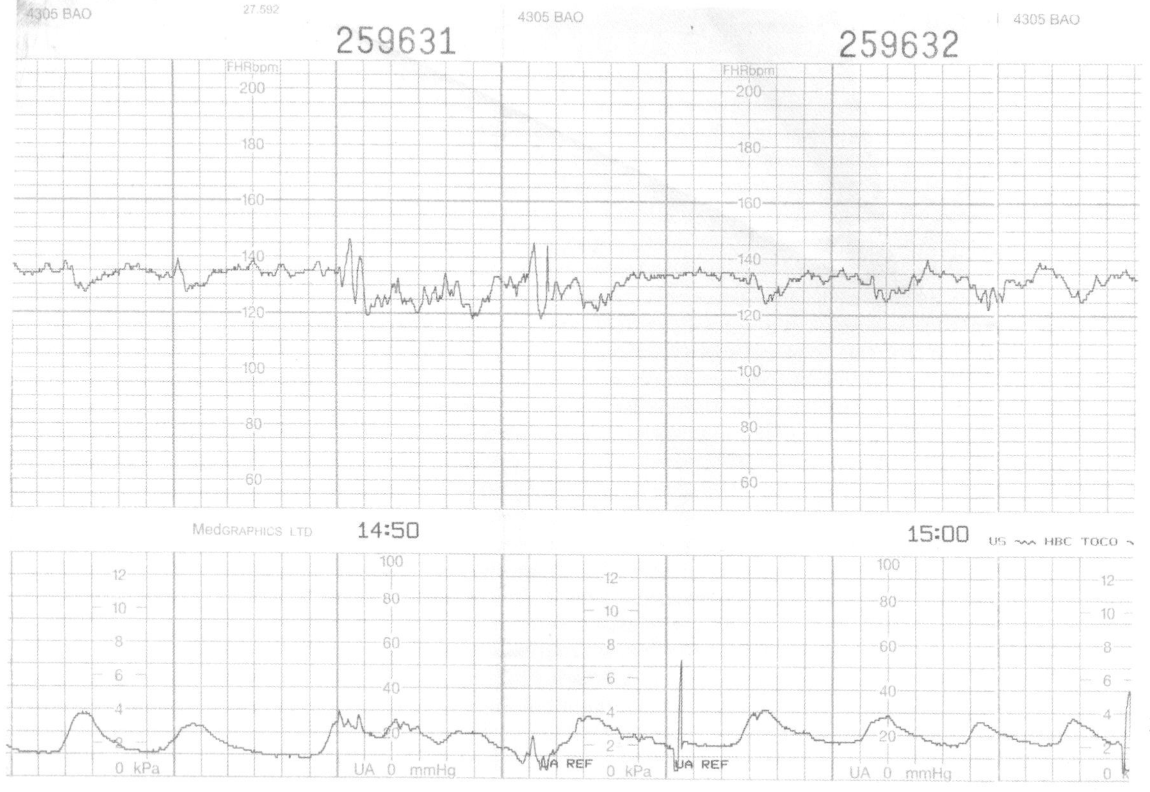

HISTORY

22-year-old gravida 1, para 0.

Past history

Normally fit and well.

Antenatal period

Developed obstetric cholestasis with raised bile acids at 38 weeks' gestation. Ultrasound scan revealed baby to be on 90th centile on customised growth chart.

Labour

Labour was induced with Prostin at 38 weeks.
Oxytocic infusion in progress, epidural maintaining good analgesia.
Vaginal examination not performed for 7 hours.
CTG (Fig. 4.21).

CTG

1. What do you notice about the baseline?
2. What do you notice about the baseline variability?
3. What periodic changes, if any, are present?
4. What do you notice about the uterine activity?
5. Would you categorise the CTG as normal/suspicious/pathological?
6. What is the most probable cause of fetal heart rate abnormality shown on this trace?
7. What treatment and/or intervention would you consider necessary for this fetal heart rate pattern?

NOTES

1

2

3

4

5

6

7

ANALYSIS

1 Baseline 135 bpm **Reassuring**
2 Variability 5–10 beats **Reassuring**
3 Early decelerations **Reassuring**
No accelerations
4 Contractions 3–4:10
5 All features are reassuring: the CTG is classified as normal. Early decelerations do not cause fetal compromise.
6 Head compression causing early decelerations.
7 Continue CTG because of oxytocic infusion. Encourage woman to be mobile or move to left lateral to ease head compression.

OUTCOME

Early decelerations continue. A fetal blood sample was performed 1 hour later. pH 7.31, base deficit 3.1 mmol/l. Normal result. The cervical os was 8 cm dilated.

Fetal blood sampling was repeated 40 minutes later as the pattern persisted. Second stage was confirmed. pH now 7.245, which is falling into the borderline category.

45 minutes later the presenting part was visible, active pushing commenced.

Normal birth 30 minutes later, with mild shoulder dystocia managed by McRoberts position.
Live girl, Apgar score 8/1 9/5. Birthweight 4.000 kg.
Cord blood analysis results within normal limits

	pH	Base deficit (mmol/l)
UA	7.1	7.9
UV	7.27	9.1

Late decelerations

SECTION 6

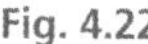

Fig. 4.22

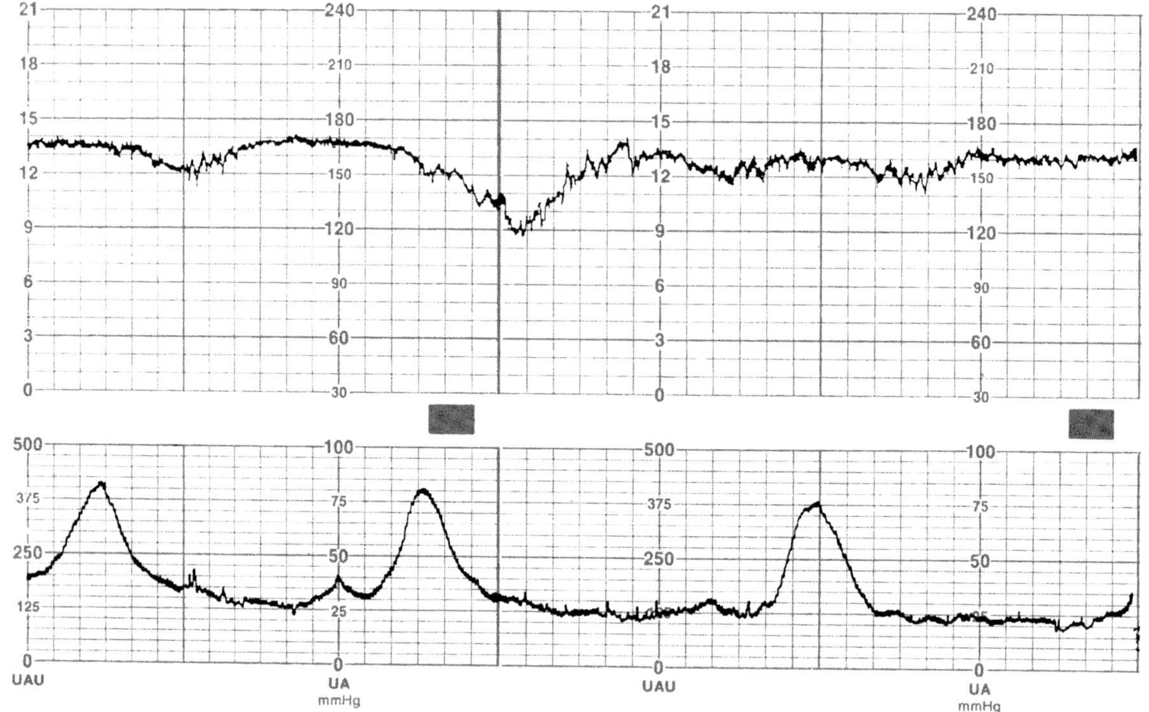

HISTORY

27-year-old gravida 1, para 0.

Past history

Nil relevant.

Antenatal period

Normal.
Admitted at 41 weeks with history of diminished fetal movements for 3 days. Mild contractions for 2 hours. Admission CTG (Fig. 4.22).

CTG

1 What do you notice about the baseline?
2 What do you notice about the baseline variability?
3 What periodic changes, if any, are present?
4 What do you notice about the uterine activity?
5 Would you categorise the CTG as normal/suspicious/pathological?
6 What is the most probable cause of fetal heart rate abnormality shown on this trace?
7 What treatment and/or intervention would you consider necessary for this fetal heart rate pattern?

NOTES

1

2

3

4

5

6

7

ANALYSIS

1	Baseline 160–165 bpm	**Non-reassuring**
2	Variability 5–10 beats	**Reassuring**
3	Late decelerations	**Abnormal**

4 Contracting 1–2 in 10 minutes.
5 There is one non-reassuring feature and one abnormal feature: the CTG is classified as pathological.
6 Late decelerations are always associated with fetal compromise. The woman has reported a change in the pattern of fetal movements over 3 days which should raise further concerns.
7 Vaginal examination to assess cervical dilation.
If cervix favourable, artificial rupture of membranes to assess the colour of the liquor and to perform fetal blood sampling.
Prepare for delivery while these actions are performed.
If cervix not favourable, deliver.

OUTCOME

24.00 hours

30 minutes after initial CTG a vaginal examination has revealed the cervical os to be 5 cm dilated.
Artificial rupture of membranes – fresh meconium-stained liquor draining.
Fetal scalp electrode applied – resulting CTG of poor quality.
Fetal blood sampling performed: pH 7.09, base excess −10 mmol/l. This result is low and warrants immediate delivery.

01.48 hours

Caesarean section performed.

Live boy.
Apgar score 4/1 8/5.
Birthweight 3.330 kg.
No cord blood samples were available.

DISCUSSION

It is important to obtain cord blood samples for analysis when there has been a concern regarding the CTG in labour, particularly if a fetal blood sample has been performed in order to confirm the diagnosis of hypoxia. The results will also assist with the management of the baby at birth.

Fig. 4.23

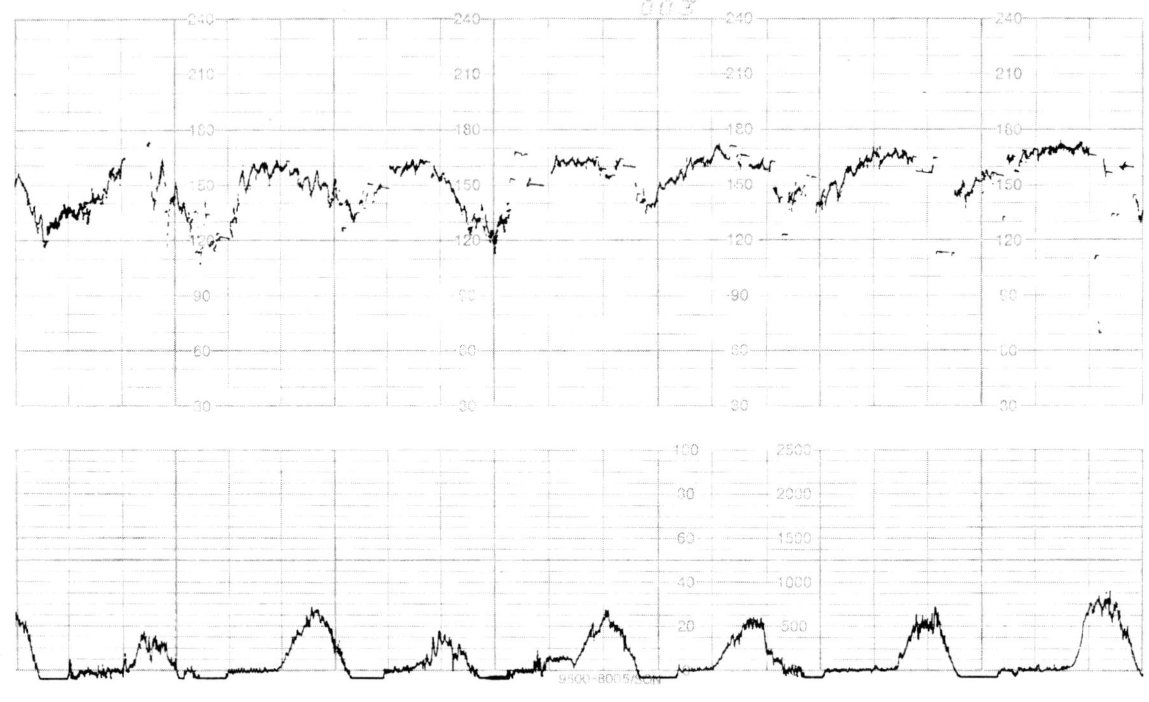

HISTORY

25-year-old gravida 1, para 0.

Past history

Nil relevant.

Antenatal period

Normal
Admitted in spontaneous labour at 41 weeks, contracting 1 in 5 minutes.

Labour

16.30 hours

Cervical os 2 cm dilated.
Artificial rupture of membrane – clear liquor draining.
Fetal scalp electrode applied.
Contractions monitored externally.

17.30 hours

CTG (Fig. 4.23).

CTG

1. What do you notice about the baseline?
2. What do you notice about the baseline variability?
3. What periodic changes, if any, are present?
4. What do you notice about the uterine activity?
5. Would you categorise the CTG as normal/suspicious/pathological?
6. What is the most probable cause of fetal heart rate abnormality shown on this trace?
7. What treatment and/or intervention would you consider necessary for this fetal heart rate pattern?

NOTES

1

2

3

4

5

6

7

ANALYSIS

1 Baseline 160–165 bpm — **Non-reassuring**
2 Variability 5 bpm — **Reassuring**
3 Late decelerations — **Abnormal**
4 Contracting 3 in 10 minutes, not adequately monitored.
5 There is one non-reassuring feature and one abnormal feature: the CTG is classified as pathological.
6 Fetal compromise must be suspected.
7 Change maternal position. Fetal blood sampling is indicated. As there is a baseline tachycardia present with decreased variability, prepare for delivery while these actions are being performed.

OUTCOME

18.00 hours

Fetal blood sampling performed: pH 7.32. This is a normal pH but no base deficit is recorded.

18.30 hours

Meconium-stained liquor noted.
Late decelerations now more prolonged.

19.00 hours

Second stage of labour diagnosed.

19.15 hours

Rotational forceps delivery.
Live boy.
Apgar score 8/1 9/5.
Birthweight 3.700 kg.
Large number of placental infarcts noted.
No cord blood samples available.

Variable decelerations

SECTION 7

Fig. 4.24

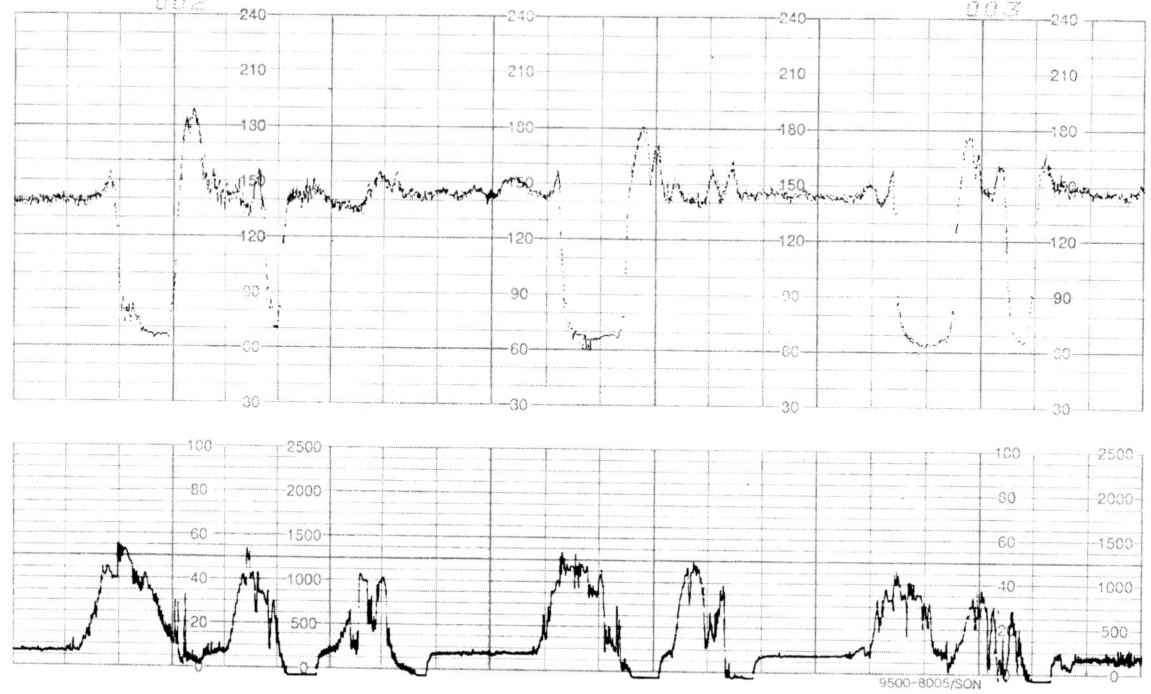

HISTORY

25-year-old gravida 1, para 0.

Past history

Nil relevant.

Antenatal period

Normal.
Admitted at 41 weeks, contracting 1 in 5 minutes.

Labour

10.30 hours

Cervical os 7 cm dilated.
Artificial rupture of membranes – clear liquor draining.
Fetal scalp electrode applied.

12.50 hours

Cervical os 8 cm dilated.
Epidural analgesia commenced.

14.30 hours

CTG (Fig. 4.24).

CTG

1 What do you notice about the baseline?
2 What do you notice about the baseline variability?
3 What periodic changes, if any, are present?
4 What do you notice about the uterine activity?
5 Would you categorise the CTG as normal/suspicious/pathological?
6 What is the most probable cause of fetal heart rate abnormality shown on this trace?
7 What treatment and/or intervention would you consider necessary for this fetal heart rate pattern?

NOTES

1

2

3

4

5

6

7

ANALYSIS

1	Baseline 140–145 bpm	**Reassuring**
2	Variability 5 bpm, some accelerations	**Reassuring**
3	Atypical variable decelerations. There is exaggerated shouldering following decelerations and they are lasting for about 1 minute	**Abnormal**
	Accelerations are also present	**Reassuring**

4 Contracting 3 in 10 minutes, varying in strength.

5 There is one abnormal feature: the CTG is classified as pathological.

6 Variable decelerations are caused by cord compression; the degree of fetal compromise that results is dependent upon the severity of the decelerations.

7 Change maternal position.
Vaginal examination to assess cervical dilation and exclude cord prolapsed. Fetal blood sampling is indicated.

OUTCOME

14.45 hours

Second stage of labour diagnosed.
Fetal blood sampling performed: pH 7.29, base excess −6 mmol/l, results within normal limits.

15.05 hours

Commenced pushing.

15.30 hours

No improvement in CTG.

15.42 hours

Straight forceps delivery.

Live girl.
Apgar score 3/1 8/5.
Birthweight 3.060 kg.
Cord around neck × 1.
No cord blood samples available.

DISCUSSION

Performing a fetal blood sample during second stage of labour gives the opportunity for a normal birth if the result is within normal limits, as in this case. It is important to bear in mind that the pH of the fetal blood drops more rapidly during the second stage, particularly with pushing; birth should not be delayed if the CTG continues to cause concern.

Fig. 4.25

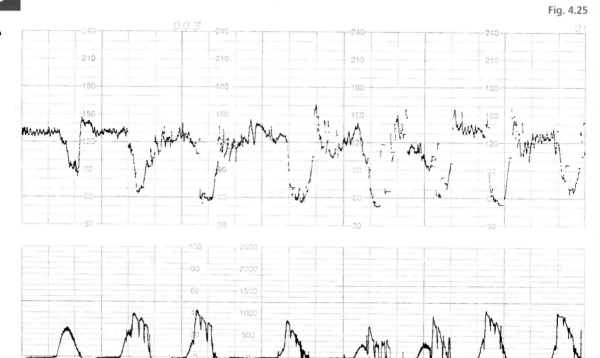

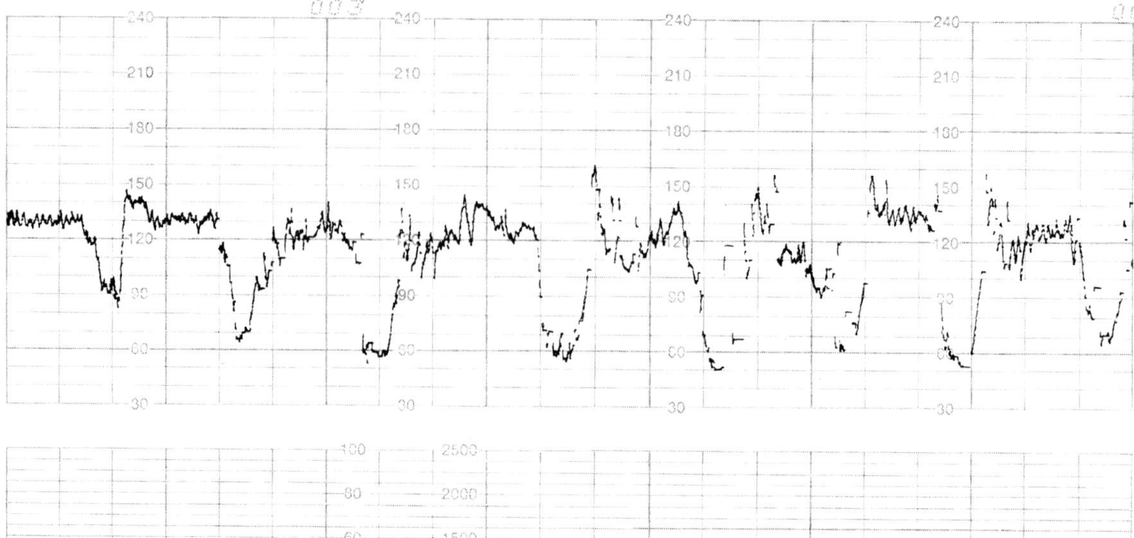

HISTORY

28-year-old gravida 1, para 0.

Past history

Nil relevant.

Antenatal period

Normal.
Admitted at 41 weeks, contracting 1 in 5 minutes, spontaneous rupture of membranes.

Labour

03.30 hours

Cervical os 4 cm dilated.
Clear liquor draining.
Fetal scalp electrode applied.
Contractions monitored externally.

04.00 hours

Epidural analgesia commenced.

05.30 hours

Second stage diagnosed.

CTG

1 What do you notice about the baseline?
2 What do you notice about the baseline variability?
3 What periodic changes, if any, are present?
4 What do you notice about the uterine activity?
5 Would you categorise the CTG as normal/suspicious/pathological?
6 What is the most probable cause of fetal heart rate abnormality shown on this trace?
7 What treatment and/or intervention would you consider necessary for this fetal heart rate pattern?

Labour continued

06.30 hours

Commenced pushing.

07.00 hours

No progress being made.
CTG (Fig. 4.25).

NOTES

1

2

3

4

5

6

7

ANALYSIS

1	Baseline 125–130 bpm	**Reassuring**
2	Variability 5–10 bpm	**Reassuring**
3	Atypical variable decelerations; there is a loss of shouldering on some of the decelerations	**Abnormal**
	Accelerations are present	**Reassuring**
4	Contracting 3–4 in 10 minutes	
5	There is one abnormal feature: the CTG is classified as pathological.	
6	Cord compression.	
7	Change maternal position. Fetal blood sampling could be considered to allow the second stage to be continued if the result is normal. In view of active pushing for over 1 hour with little progress it is appropriate to consider expediting birth.	

OUTCOME

07.40 hours

Straight forceps delivery.
Live girl.
Apgar score 9/1 9/5.
Birthweight 2.840 kg.
Cord around neck × 1.

Fig. 4.26

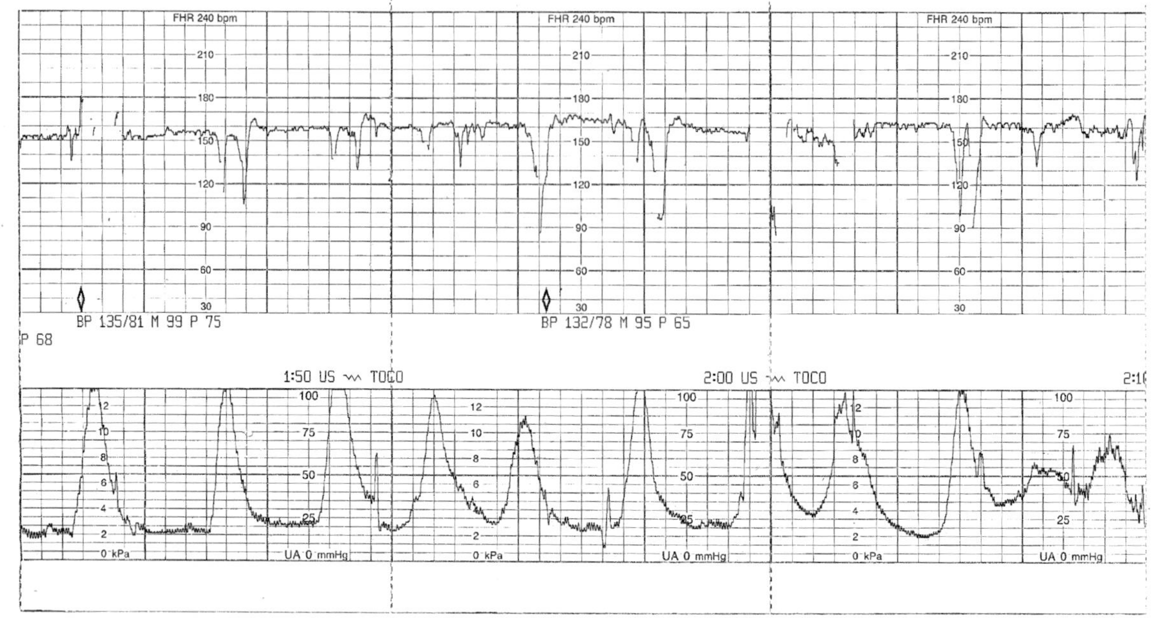

HISTORY

27-year-old gravida 1, para 0.

Past history

Nil relevant.

Antenatal period

Subchorionic bleed noted at 29 weeks on ultrasound scan.
Follow-up scans normal, growth good.
Pregnancy progressed well.
Admitted at term plus 11 days for surgical induction of labour.

Labour

10.00 hours

Artificial rupture of membranes – clear liquor draining.
Initial external CTG normal.

10.45 hours

Syntocinon (oxytocin) infusion commenced.
Continuous external CTG commenced.

16.30 hours

Epidural analgesia in progress.
CTG normal.

CTG

1 What do you notice about the baseline?
2 What do you notice about the baseline variability?
3 What periodic changes, if any, are present?
4 What do you notice about the uterine activity?
5 Would you categorise the CTG as normal/suspicious/pathological?
6 What is the most probable cause of fetal heart rate abnormality shown on this trace?
7 What treatment and/or intervention would you consider necessary for this fetal heart rate pattern?

Labour continued

01.15 hours

Cervical os 7 cm dilated, clear liquor draining.
Progress in labour slow.

01.50 hours

CTG (Fig. 4.26).

NOTES

1

2

3

4

5

6

7

ANALYSIS

1 Baseline 155–160 bpm — **Reassuring**
2 Variability less than 5, no accelerations — **Non-reassuring**
3 Atypical variable decelerations, loss of shouldering — **Abnormal**
4 Contracting 3–4 in 10 minutes.
5 There is one non-reassuring and one abnormal feature: the CTG is classified as pathological.
6 Cord compression: the degree of compromise is difficult to ascertain. Variability may be reduced as a result of a fetal sleep pattern but may be a sign of compromise.
7 Change maternal position.
Record maternal temperature and pulse rate.
Fetal blood sampling is indicated as it is a pathological CTG.

OUTCOME

Woman apyrexial, pulse rate 92 bpm.
Variable decelerations reduce, occasional typical variable decelerations only.

05.00 hours

Progressed to second stage of labour.

06.50 hours

No progress made with maternal effort.
Cephalic presentation still one-fifth palpable abdominally.
Occasional typical variable decelerations continue.
Emergency caesarean section performed.
Live boy.
Apgar score 9/1 9/5.
Birthweight 3.840 kg.
Cord gases: pH 7.40, base excess –3.2 mmol/l: this is a normal result but only one vessel has been sampled. It is not possible to know which one it is; therefore a degree of acidaemia cannot be ruled out. It is important that both vessels are sampled for an accurate result.

Fig. 4.27

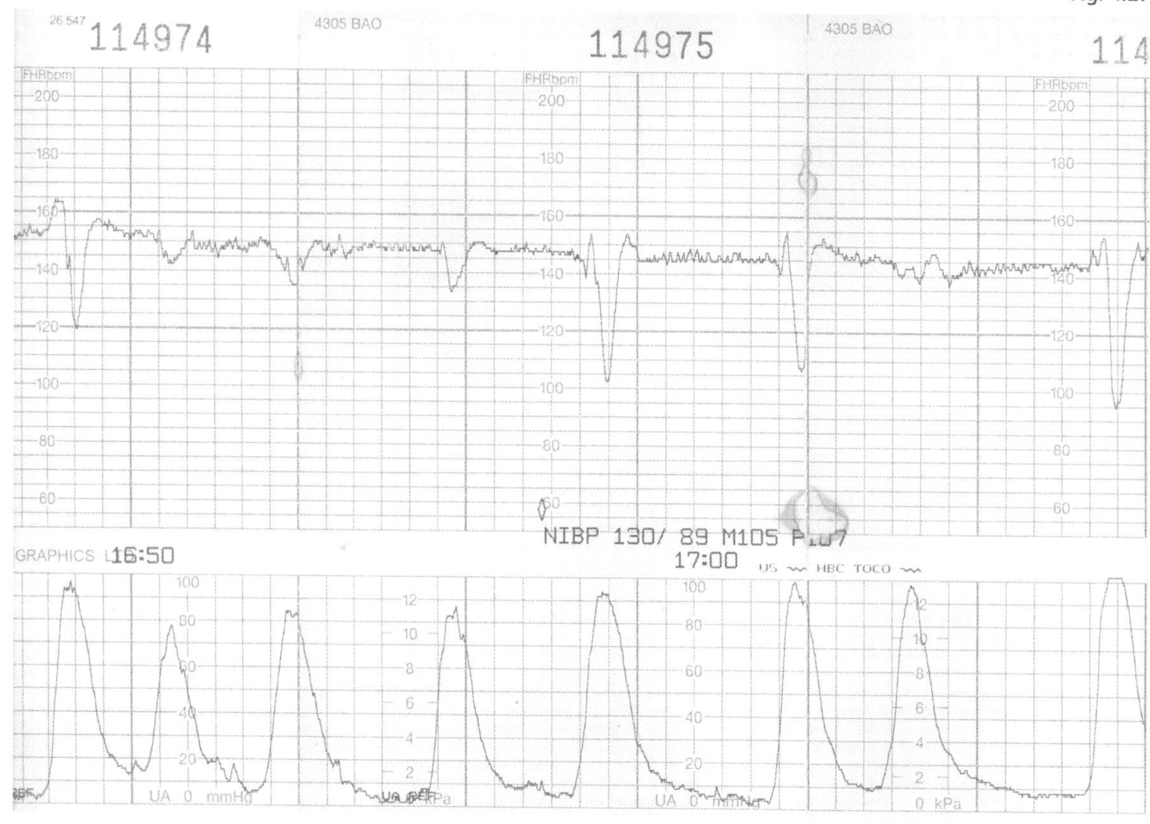

HISTORY

27-year-old gravida 2, para 0 + 1.

Past history

Nil relevant.

Antenatal period

No problems identified. Low risk, midwife-led care.

Labour

Admitted at 40 + 5 in spontaneous labour. Cervix thin, os 3 cm dilated on vaginal examination. Mobilising. Membranes ruptured 2 hours later, clear liquor draining, continues to mobilise, no analgesia. Fetal heart rate monitored by intermittent auscultation, no abnormalities heard.
4 hours later, requesting analgesia. Vaginal examination performed, no change in cervical dilatation. Oxytocic infusion and continuous external fetal heart rate monitoring commenced.
CTG (Fig. 4.27).

CTG

1 What do you notice about the baseline?
2 What do you notice about the baseline variability?
3 What periodic changes, if any, are present?
4 What do you notice about the uterine activity?
5 Would you categorise the CTG as normal/suspicious/pathological?
6 What is the most probable cause of fetal heart rate abnormality shown on this trace?
7 What treatment and/or intervention would you consider necessary for this fetal heart rate pattern?

NOTES

1

2

3

4

5

6

7

ANALYSIS

1 Baseline 145 bpm — **Reassuring**
2 Variability 5 beats — **Reassuring**
3 Typical variable decelerations — **Non-reassuring**
No accelerations
4 Contracting 3–4 in 10 minutes.
5 There is one non-reassuring feature: the CTG is classified as suspicious.
6 Cord compression: at present the decelerations are quick to recover to baseline.
7 Change maternal position. Continue to observe CTG.

OUTCOME

2 hours later, occasional typical variable decelerations continue. Repeat vaginal examination shows no further cervical dilatation. Decision made for caesarean section. Live boy. Apgar score 9/1 10/5. Birthweight 3.330 kg.

Cord blood analysis results within normal limits.

	pH	Base deficit (mmol/l)
UA	7.24	3.0
UV	7.2	3.0

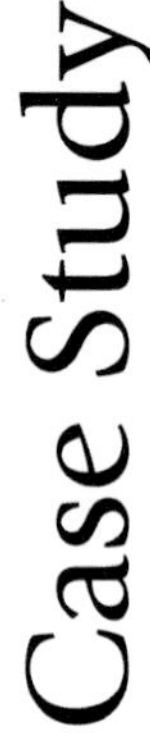

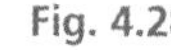

Fig. 4.28

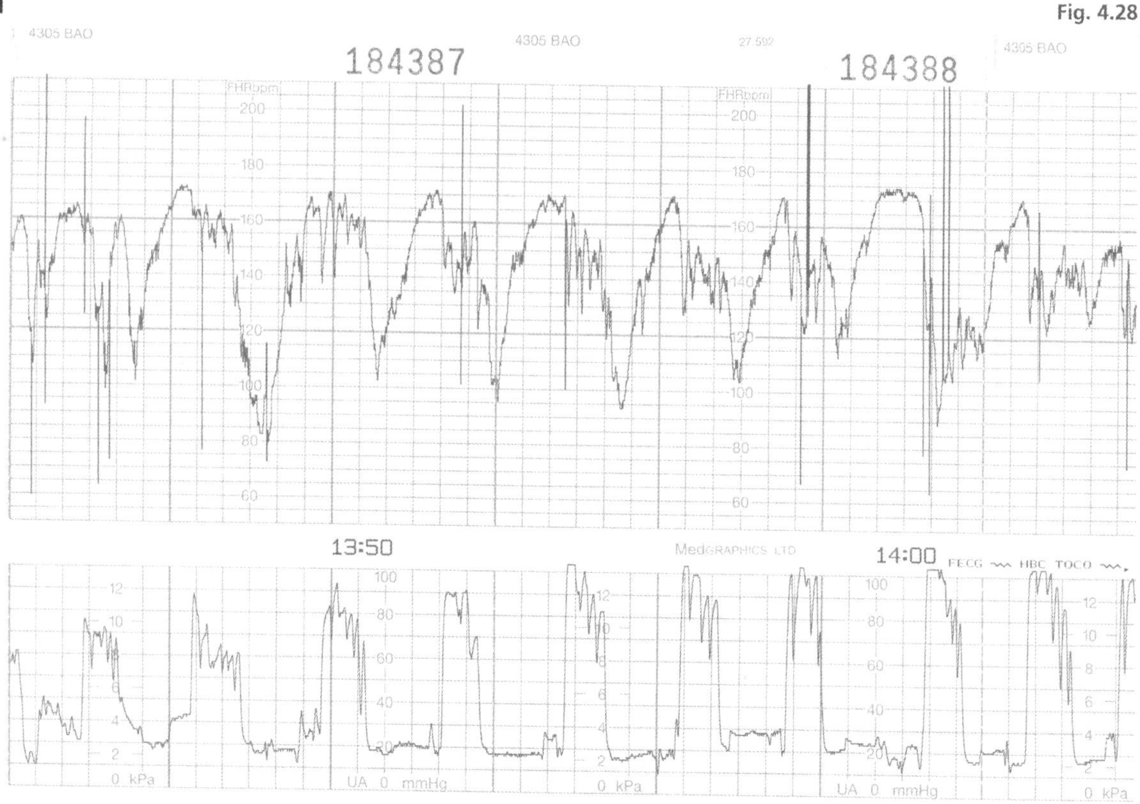

HISTORY

32-year-old gravida 6, para 4 + 1.

Past history

Previous caesarean section for breech presentation. Two normal births since.

Antenatal period

Well throughout. Cephalic presentation, for vaginal birth.

Labour

Admitted at 39 + 5 with spontaneous rupture of membranes, clear liquor draining, fetal movements normal. Contractions mild and irregular. Admission CTG in view of previous normal caesarean section. Admitted to await established labour.

Five hours later contractions now 4:10, atypical variable decelerations on CTG, all other features reassuring. Vaginal examination: cervical os 9 cm dilated. Fetal blood sampling performed. pH 7.27, base deficit 5.2 mmol/l, normal result.

10 minutes later commenced active pushing.
CTG (Fig. 4.28).

CTG

1. What do you notice about the baseline?
2. What do you notice about the baseline variability?
3. What periodic changes, if any, are present?
4. What do you notice about the uterine activity?
5. Would you categorise the CTG as normal/suspicious/pathological?
6. What is the most probable cause of fetal heart rate abnormality shown on this trace?
7. What treatment and/or intervention would you consider necessary for this fetal heart rate pattern?

NOTES

1

2

3

4

5

6

7

ANALYSIS

1 Baseline 160–170 bpm **Non-reassuring**
2 Variability 5–10 beats **Reassuring**
3 Atypical variable decelerations **Abnormal**
No accelerations
4 Contracting 3–4 in 10 minutes, pushing.
5 There is one non-reassuring feature and one abnormal feature: the CTG is classified as pathological.
6 Cord compression will cause variable decelerations. The increased baseline could be an indicator of fetal compromise. Alternatively this may not be a tachycardic baseline but exaggerated shouldering on the decelerations. There are some areas where the baseline is possible, showing at about 140 bpm. Because there is little rest between the contractions it is difficult to be sure.
7 Change maternal position. Fetal blood sampling is indicated, particularly if progress in second stage is of concern. The pH of the baby's blood drops quickly in the second stage, even more so with active pushing. The result will give an indication if normal birth can proceed or if assisted birth should be suggested.

OUTCOME

Fetal blood sampling was performed. pH 7.26, base deficit 5.0 mmol/l – normal results. Pushing continued for 10 minutes. No further progress was made. Birth was expedited by vacuum extraction. Live girl, Apgar score 7/1 9/5, birthweight 3.000 kg.

Cord gases, only UV available.

pH 7.23, base deficit 2.3 mmol/l.

Acidaemia cannot be ruled out as there is only a venous sample result.

Fig. 4.29

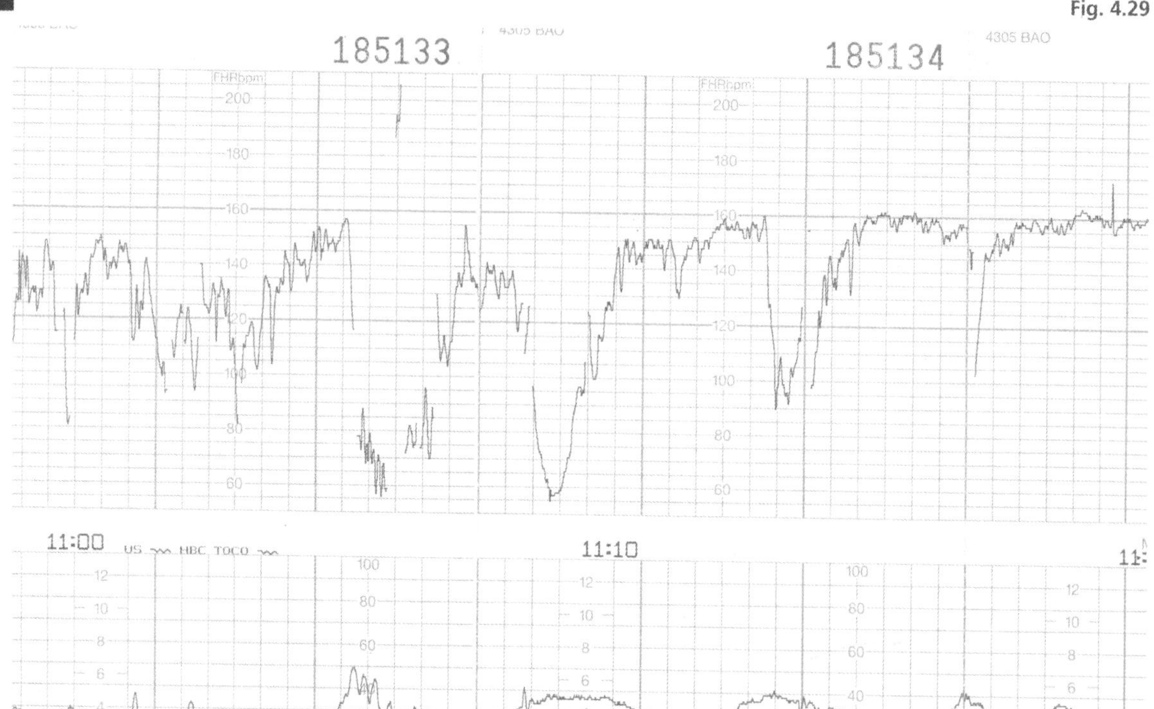

HISTORY

36-year-old gravida 1, para 0.

Past history

Epileptic on medication. No fits for many years.

Antenatal period

Well, no problems identified. Remained seizure-free. Baby on 90th centile on serial symphysiofundal height measurements.

Labour

Admitted at 39 weeks in spontaneous labour. Cervical os 5 cm dilated. Fetal heart rate auscultated at 142 bpm. Spontaneous rupture of membranes 2 hours later, clear liquor draining. 30 minutes later, deceleration heard on auscultation. CTG commenced, vaginal examination performed, cervical os 9 cm dilated.

Fetal blood sample was obtained. pH 7.29, base excess 3.4 mmol/l, normal result.
CTG (Fig. 4.29).

CTG

1 What do you notice about the baseline?
2 What do you notice about the baseline variability?
3 What periodic changes, if any, are present?
4 What do you notice about the uterine activity?
5 Would you categorise the CTG as normal/suspicious/pathological?
6 What is the most probable cause of fetal heart rate abnormality shown on this trace?
7 What treatment and/or intervention would you consider necessary for this fetal heart rate pattern?

NOTES

1

2

3

4

5

6

7

ANALYSIS

1	Baseline 155–160 bpm	**Reassuring**
2	Variability 5–10 beats	**Reassuring**
3	Atypical variable decelerations, loss of shouldering, deep deceleration with longer recovery time No accelerations	**Abnormal**

4 Contracting 3:10 minutes, not monitored adequately.
5 There is one abnormal feature: the CTG is classified as pathological.
6 Cord compression will cause variable decelerations. Ongoing atypical variables are associated with fetal compromise.
7 Change maternal position. Fetal blood sampling should be repeated in 1 hour if the pattern persists or sooner if other non-reassuring features appear.

OUTCOME

Second stage of labour diagnosed shortly after CTG sample. Decelerations became deeper and longer-lasting, birth not imminent. Straight forceps delivery, live boy, Apgar score 8/1 9/5, birthweight 4.160 kg.

Cord blood analysis results within normal limits.

	pH	Base deficit (mmol/l)
UA	7.12	8
UV	7.21	8.3

Results do not demonstrate evidence of acidaemia.

DISCUSSION

Typical variable decelerations demonstrate a normal response to cord compression. Most babies will tolerate the resultant reduction in oxygenated blood and the other features of the CTG will remain normal. The development of atypical variables indicates that the baby is not adapting to the reduction in oxygenation as well and is possibly developing hypoxia. In addition other features may be changing. In this instance there is an increase in baseline rate during the course of the CTG and variability, although just within normal limits, has reduced. The decelerations are also dropping to around 60 bpm; this can affect cardiac function, which increases the risk of hypoxia. Once pushing commences, which further decreases oxygen transfer, the variable decelerations worsen and expedition of birth is deemed to be the safest course of action.

Prolonged decelerations

SECTION 8

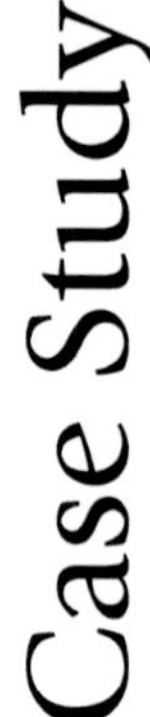

Fig. 4.30

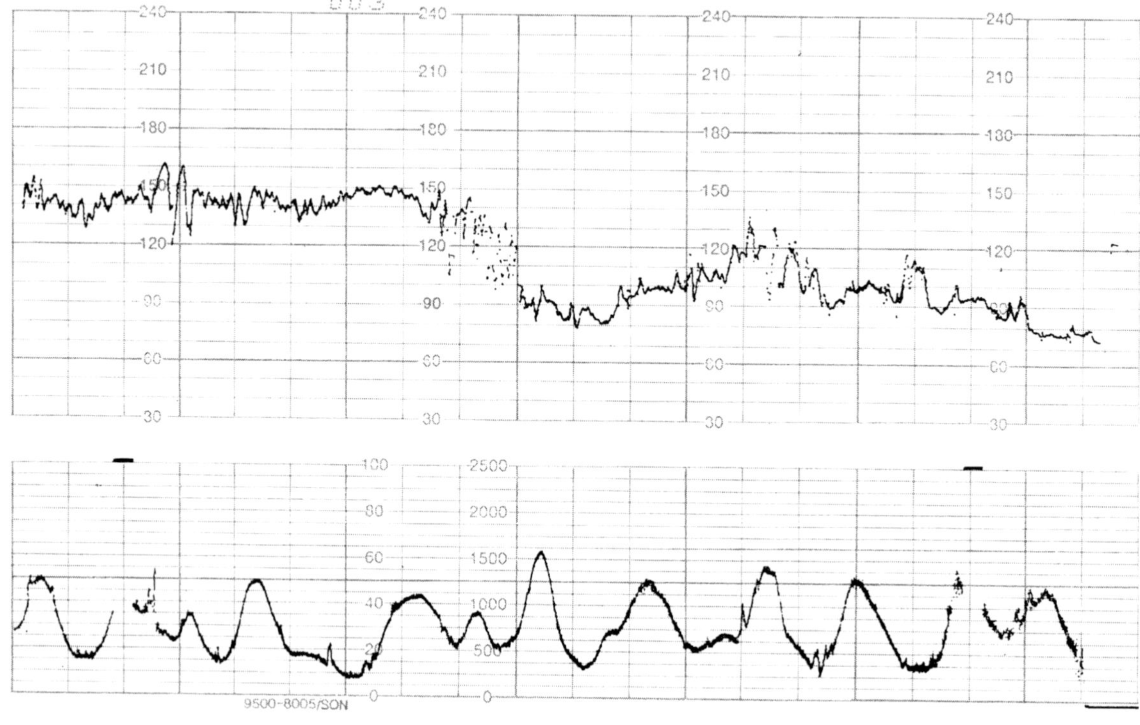

HISTORY

23-year-old gravida 2, para 0 + 1.

Past history

Nil relevant.

Antenatal period

Normal
Admitted at 41 weeks with spontaneous rupture of membranes – slightly meconium-stained liquor draining.

Labour

21.40 hours

Cervical os 4 cm dilated.
Fetal scalp electrode applied.
Contractions monitored externally.

22.20 hours

Epidural analgesia commenced.

23.15 hours

Cervical os 6 cm dilated.

Labour continued

23.30 hours

Epidural top-up given.

24.00 hours

Occasional typical variable decelerations noted.

00.50 hours

CTG (Fig. 4.30).

CTG

1 What do you notice about the baseline?
2 What do you notice about the baseline variability?
3 What periodic changes, if any, are present?
4 What do you notice about the uterine activity?
5 Would you categorise the CTG as normal/suspicious/pathological?
6 What is the most probable cause of fetal heart rate abnormality shown on this trace?
7 What treatment and/or intervention would you consider necessary for this fetal heart rate pattern?

NOTES

1

2

3

4

5

6

7

ANALYSIS

1 Baseline 120 bpm — **Reassuring**
2 Variability 5 beats — **Reassuring**
3 Prolonged deceleration lasting 7 minutes — **Abnormal**
4 Contracting 4–5 in 10 minutes, varying in strength.
5 One abnormal feature: the CTG is classified as pathological.
6 Previous variable decelerations – cord compression or total occlusion possible. Epidural top-up was given 50 minutes ago so unlikely to be hypotension but should be borne in mind.
7 Vaginal examination to assess cervical dilation and to exclude cord prolapse.
Change maternal position.
Record blood pressure, correct with intravenous fluids if hypotensive.
As the bradycardia has lasted for 7 minutes, urgent preparations should be made for delivery by caesarean section if cervix not fully dilated or if vaginal birth deemed to be difficult. The fetal heart rate should be auscultated prior to surgery and if the rate is normal, the CTG recommenced. If the baseline rate has recovered then fetal blood sampling should be performed. If normal, labour could be allowed to continue; otherwise operative delivery should proceed.

OUTCOME

Cervical os 8 cm dilated.
No cord prolapse.
Fetal blood sampling attempted – failed.
Fetal heart returned to baseline 120–130 bpm, with occasional typical variable decelerations.

03.33 hours

Second stage of labour diagnosed.

04.15 hours

Normal birth.
Live boy.
Apgar score 1/1 7/5.
Birthweight 3.140 kg.
No cord blood sample available.
True knot in cord.

Complex

SECTION 9

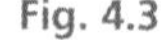

Fig. 4.31

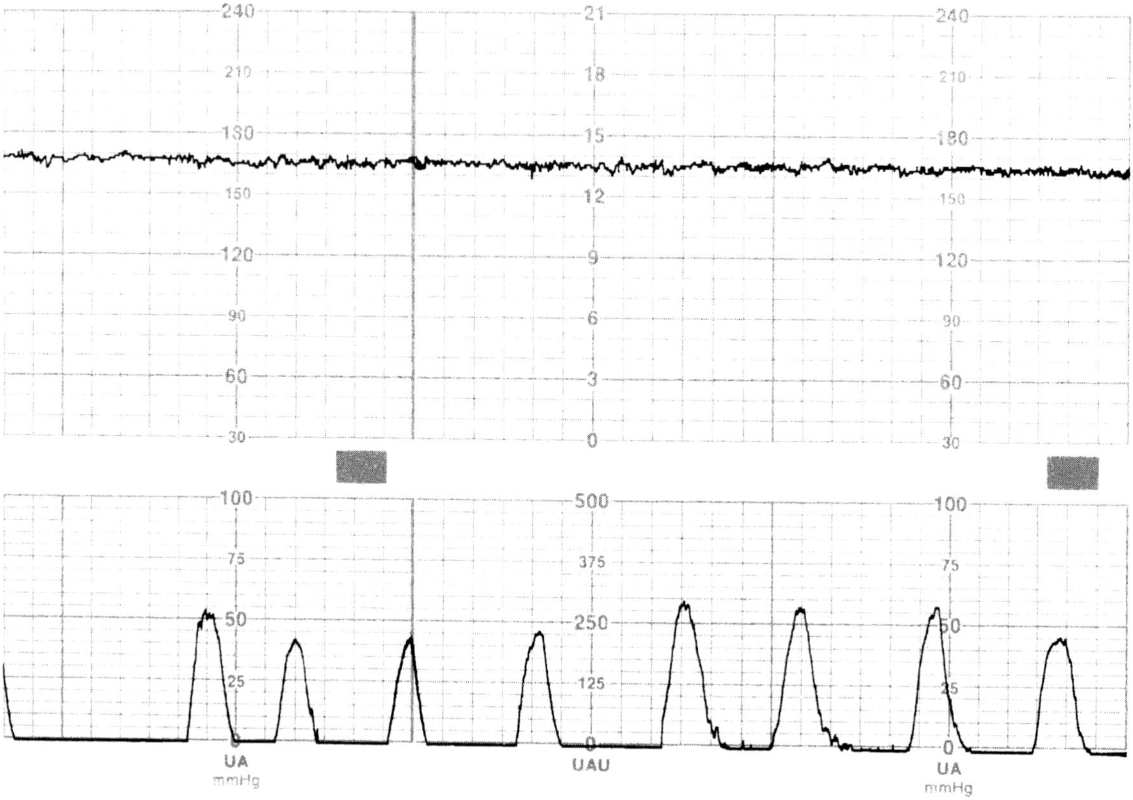

HISTORY

29-year-old gravida 1, para 0.

Past history

Nil relevant.

Antenatal period

Admitted at 39 weeks, history of diminished fetal movements for 3 days.
Admission CTG (Fig. 4.31).

CTG

1. What do you notice about the baseline?
2. What do you notice about the baseline variability?
3. What periodic changes, if any, are present?
4. What do you notice about the uterine activity?
5. Would you categorise the CTG as normal/suspicious/pathological?
6. What is the most probable cause of fetal heart rate abnormality shown on this trace?
7. What treatment and/or intervention would you consider necessary for this fetal heart rate pattern?

NOTES

1

2

3

4

5

6

7

ANALYSIS

1 Baseline 165 bpm — **Non-reassuring**
2 Variability less than 5 beats — **Non-reassuring**
3 No decelerations — **Reassuring**
No accelerations — **? Significance**
4 Tightening 4–5 in 10 minutes, not painful.
5 There are two non-reassuring features: the CTG is classified as pathological.
6 Fetal sleep pattern may explain the reduction in variability. The baseline is slightly raised above 160 bpm. However there is a history of a change in the pattern of fetal movements for 3 days, which may indicate fetal compromise. The fetal heart rate abnormalities are present in the absence of contractions; although uterine activity is displayed on the CTG, the woman is not aware of it.
7 Change maternal position.
Vaginal examination to assess cervical dilation, with a view to performing artificial rupture of membranes to observe colour of the liquor.
Prepare for delivery if the cervix is not favourable.

OUTCOME

Cervix posterior, 1 cm long, os 0.5 cm dilated.
Caesarean section performed.
Live girl.
Apgar score 1/1 5/5.
Birthweight 2.980 kg.
No cord blood sample available.
Thick, fresh meconium noted at delivery.
Baby transferred to neonatal unit.
Listeriosis diagnosed at 2 days old; subsequently recovered and discharged home.

DISCUSSION

Whilst fetal sleep is an explanation for reduced variability it is important that all features of the CTG along with the history that the woman gives are taken into consideration before making a decision on the interpretation of the CTG. When CTG abnormalities are present and the woman gives a history of altered pattern of fetal movements, bleeding per vaginam or abdominal pain, then there is an indication to continue the CTG for a longer period until the features return to a reassuring pattern.

Fig. 4.32

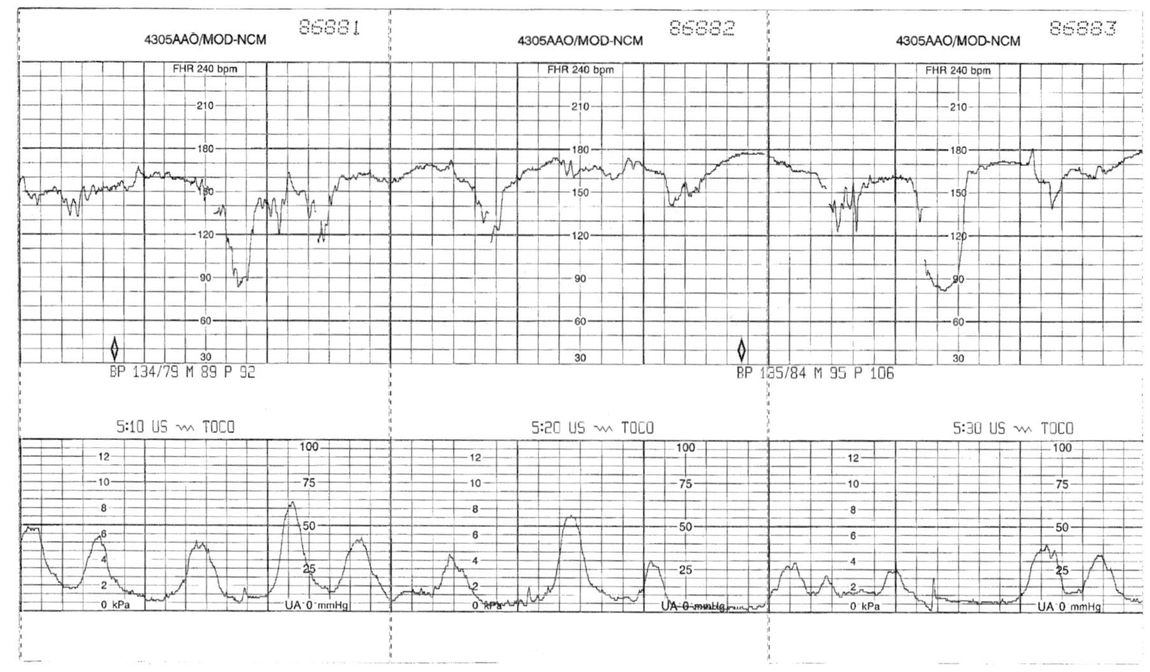

HISTORY

28-year-old gravida 1, para 0.

Past history

Nil relevant.

Antenatal period

Mild hypertension from 36 weeks.
No proteinurea.
Prostin induction of labour at 39 weeks' gestation.

Labour

04.00 hours

Cervical os 4 cm dilated.
Artificial rupture of membranes performed – clear liquor draining.
Epidural analgesia commenced.
Continuous external fetal monitoring in progress.

05.10 hours

CTG (Fig. 4.32).

CTG

1 What do you notice about the baseline?
2 What do you notice about the baseline variability?
3 What periodic changes, if any, are present?
4 What do you notice about the uterine activity?
5 Would you categorise the CTG as normal/suspicious/pathological?
6 What is the most probable cause of fetal heart rate abnormality shown on this trace?
7 What treatment and/or intervention would you consider necessary for this fetal heart rate pattern?

NOTES

1

2

3

4

5

6

7

ANALYSIS

1 Baseline initially 160 bpm rising to 180 bpm **Non-reassuring**
2 Variability less than 5 beats **Non-reassuring**
3 Atypical variable decelerations, loss of shouldering **Abnormal**
4 Contracting 3–4 in 10 minutes, irregular in strength and frequency.
5 There are two non-reassuring and one abnormal feature: the CTG is classified as pathological.
6 Cord compression will result in atypical variable decelerations, but will not explain the tachycardia or reduction in variability. These could be explained by fetal compromise developed as a result of the degree of cord compression. It is worth bearing in mind fetal sleep pattern in which case normal variability should be apparent within 90 minutes. Fetal tachycardia may be due to maternal pyrexia.
This is a complex CTG with a number of abnormalities. Fetal compromise must be excluded. Even though all three concerning features potentially have their own explanations when seen together it is far more worrying.
7 Record maternal temperature. Change maternal position. Discontinue any oxytocic infusion. Fetal blood sampling should be performed.

OUTCOME

Maternal temperature 37.5 °C.
Variable decelerations persist, with tachycardia; variability improves.

06.10 hours

Fetal blood sampling performed: pH 7.34, base deficit 3.6 mmol/l, normal result.

09.00 hours

Cervical os 8–9 cm dilated.

09.30 hours

Maternal temperature now 36.8 °C.
CTG as before.
Repeat fetal blood sampling performed: pH 7.37, base deficit 3.1 mmol/l, normal result.

10.15 hours

Cervical os 8 cm dilated, therefore decision made for emergency caesarean section based on progress in labour.
Live girl.
Apgar score 7/1 9/5.
Birthweight 3.320 kg.
Cord blood analysis result only from one vessel, therefore unable to rule out acidaemia accurately.
pH 7.34, base deficit 2.7 mmol/l.

DISCUSSION

The role of fetal blood sampling in this case demonstrates how, despite a pathological CTG with normal blood gases, the labour was allowed to progress with the potential for a normal birth. It is unfortunate that this did not occur and caesarean section was necessary. Cord blood results from both vessels would also have justified the decision to allow labour to progress.

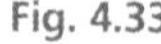
Fig. 4.33

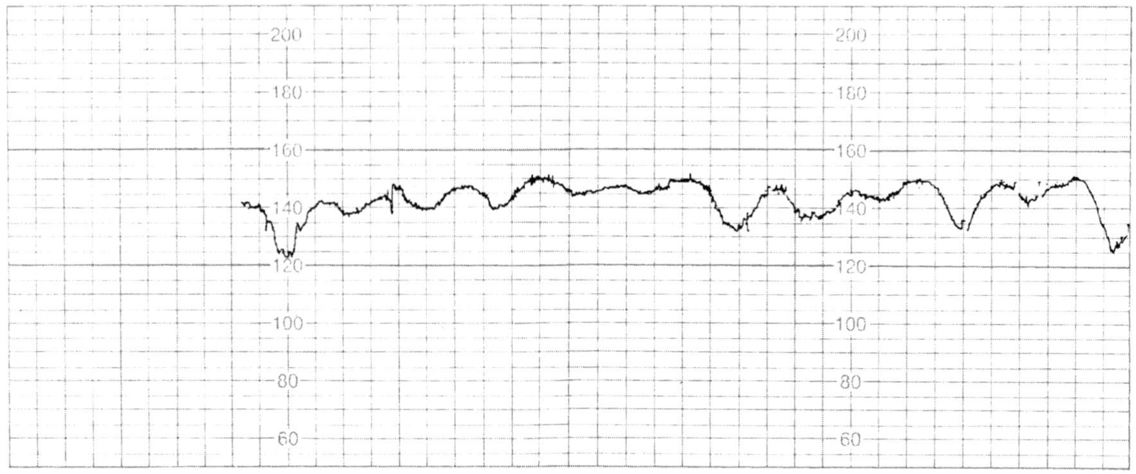

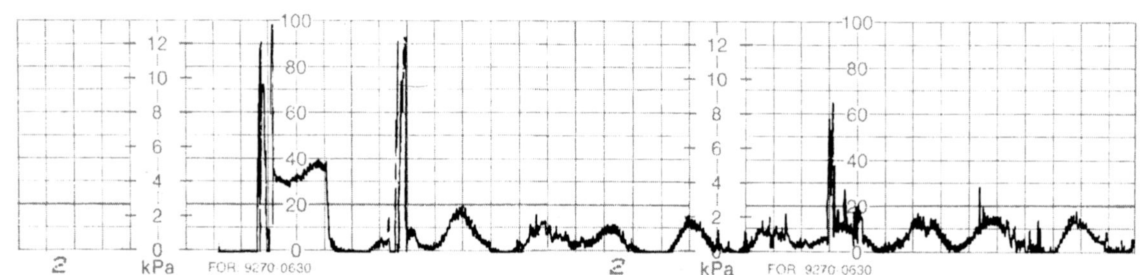

HISTORY

18-year-old gravida 1, para 0.

Past history

Nil relevant.

Antenatal period

Normal.
Admitted at 36 weeks with history of heavy, fresh bleeding per vaginam for 2 hours, of sudden onset; complaining of abdominal pain.
On examination: abdomen tense and tender; moderate amount of fresh bleeding per vaginam.
Admission CTG (Fig. 4.33).

CTG

1. What do you notice about the baseline?
2. What do you notice about the baseline variability?
3. What periodic changes, if any, are present?
4. What do you notice about the uterine activity?
5. Would you categorise this CTG as normal/suspicious/patyhological?
6. What is the most probable cause of fetal heart rate abnormality shown on this trace?
7. What treatment and/or intervention would you consider necessary for this fetal heart rate pattern?

NOTES

1

2

3

4

5

6

7

ANALYSIS

1 Baseline 145–150 bpm — **Reassuring**
2 Variability virtually absent — **Non-reassuring**
3 Late decelerations — **Abnormal**
4 Uterine irritability.
5 There is one abnormal and one reassuring feature: the CTG is classified as pathological.
6 Reduced placental blood flow due to placental abruption – fetal hypoxia.
7 Prepare for immediate delivery. Change maternal position.

OUTCOME

Ultrasound scan performed – posterior upper-segment placenta.
On vaginal examination the cervix 1 cm long, cervical os 2 cm dilated.
Caesarean section performed.
Baby girl.
Apgar score 0/1 7/5 9/10.
No cord blood sample available.
Resuscitated successfully.
Birthweight 2.690 kg.
Couvelaire uterus noted.
Baby discharged home at 3 weeks, well.

DISCUSSION

Variability of less than 5 beats for 40–90 minutes is a non-reassuring feature and would place a CTG in a suspicious category. Once this has persisted for longer than 90 minutes, the feature becomes abnormal and the category changes to pathological.

It must be emphasised that it is not deemed acceptable to wait for 90 minutes before taking further actions without taking into account the clinical situation. In this case it was obvious that a large antepartum haemorrhage had occurred, the CTG is grossly abnormal and delivery of the baby needed to be expedited.

Fig. 4.34

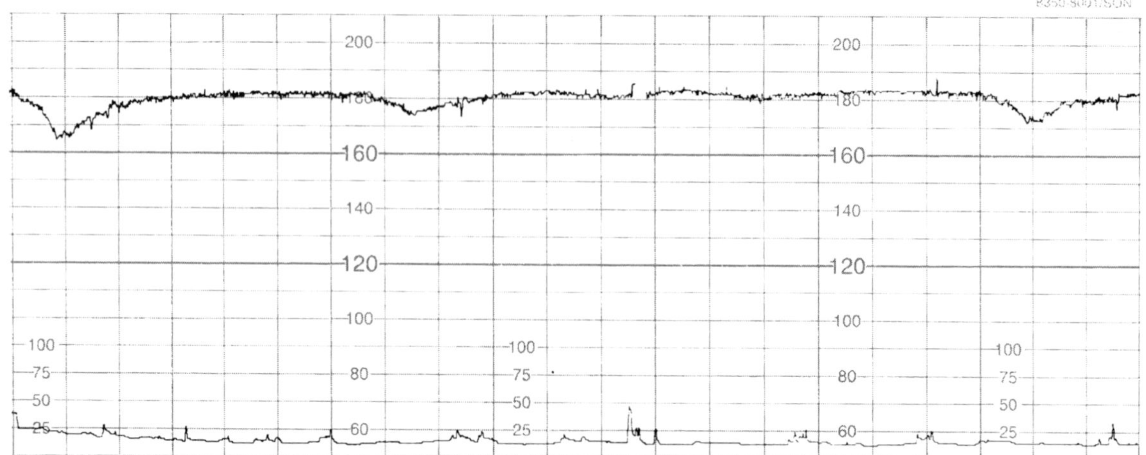

HISTORY

36-year-old gravida 3, para 2.

Past history

Nil relevant.

Antenatal period

Admitted at 33 weeks with raised blood pressure.
Diminished fetal movements.
Ultrasound scan shows asymmetrical growth retardation and reduced liquor volume.
Admission CTG (Fig. 4.34).

CTG

1 What do you notice about the baseline?
2 What do you notice about the baseline variability?
3 What periodic changes, if any, are present?
4 What do you notice about the uterine activity?
5 Would you categorise the CTG as normal/suspicious/pathological?
6 What is the most probable cause of fetal heart rate abnormality shown on this trace?
7 What treatment and/or intervention would you consider necessary for this fetal heart rate pattern?

NOTES

1

2

3

4

5

6

7

ANALYSIS

1 Baseline 180 bpm **Non-reassuring**
2 Variability appears to be virtually absent **Non-reassuring**
3 Shallow decelerations, cannot be classified in absence of contractions, unprovoked antenatal decelerations **Abnormal**
4 No contractions.
5 There is one abnormal and two non-reassuring features: the CTG is classified as pathological.
6 History of intrauterine growth retardation, diminished liquor volume, diminished fetal movements, fetal tachycardia, decreased variability, decelerations occurring without contractions – fetal compromise.
7 Prepare for delivery.

OUTCOME

Emergency caesarean section performed.
Live boy.
Apgar score 1/1 4/5 8/10, birthweight 1.470 kg.
No cord blood sample available.
True knot in cord.
Baby transferred to neonatal unit.
Discharged home at 4 weeks, well.

Fig. 4.35, Part 1 *Routine CTG.*

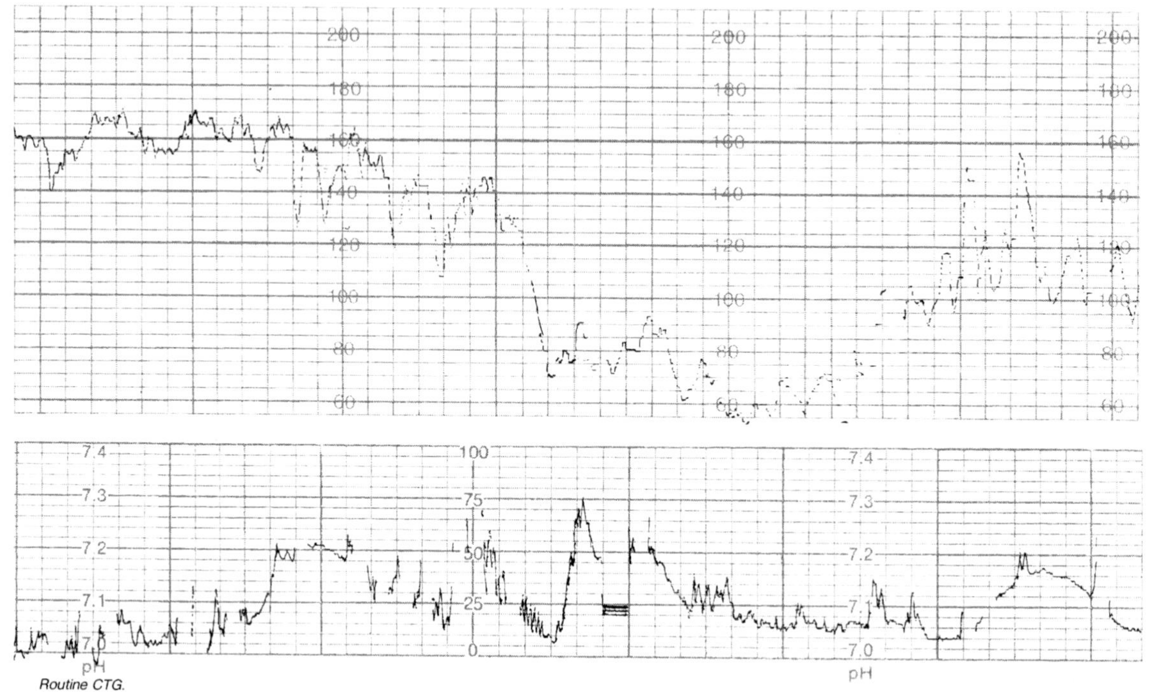

HISTORY

27-year-old gravida 2, para 1.

Past history

Nil relevant.

Antenatal period

Normal.
Admitted at 43 weeks for routine CTG (Fig. 4.35, part 1).

CTG

1 What do you notice about the baseline?
2 What do you notice about the baseline variability?
3 What periodic changes, if any, are present?
4 What do you notice about the uterine activity?
5 Would you categorise the CTG as normal/suspicious/pathological?
6 What is the most probable cause of fetal heart rate abnormality shown on this trace?
7 What treatment and/or intervention would you consider necessary for this fetal heart rate pattern?

NOTES

1

2

3

4

5

6

7

ANALYSIS

1 Baseline 150–160 bpm **Reassuring**
2 Variability 5–10 beats **Reassuring**
3 Prolonged deceleration lasting over 3 minutes with slow recovery to baseline **Abnormal**
4 Occasional tightening, no contractions.
5 There is one abnormal feature: the CTG is classified as pathological.
6 Cord occlusion is a possibility.
Note gestation; placental insufficiency resulting in fetal hypoxia must be considered.
7 Prepare for delivery.
Vaginal examination to assess cervix. If deceleration recovers and cervix favourable, consider surgical induction of labour.

OUTCOME

15.00 hours

Surgical induction of labour performed.
Cervix 1.5 cm long, cervical os 3 cm dilated.
Artificial rupture of membranes – fresh meconium-stained liquor draining.
Fetal scalp electrode applied.
Contractions monitored externally.
Contracting spontaneously.

15.45 hours

Pethidine 100 mg and Sparine 25 mg given intramuscularly.

16.00 hours

CTG – see Part 2, pages 11–25.

Case 35 continued over page.

Case 35 continued

Fig. 4.35 Part 2 *CTG at 16.00 hours.*

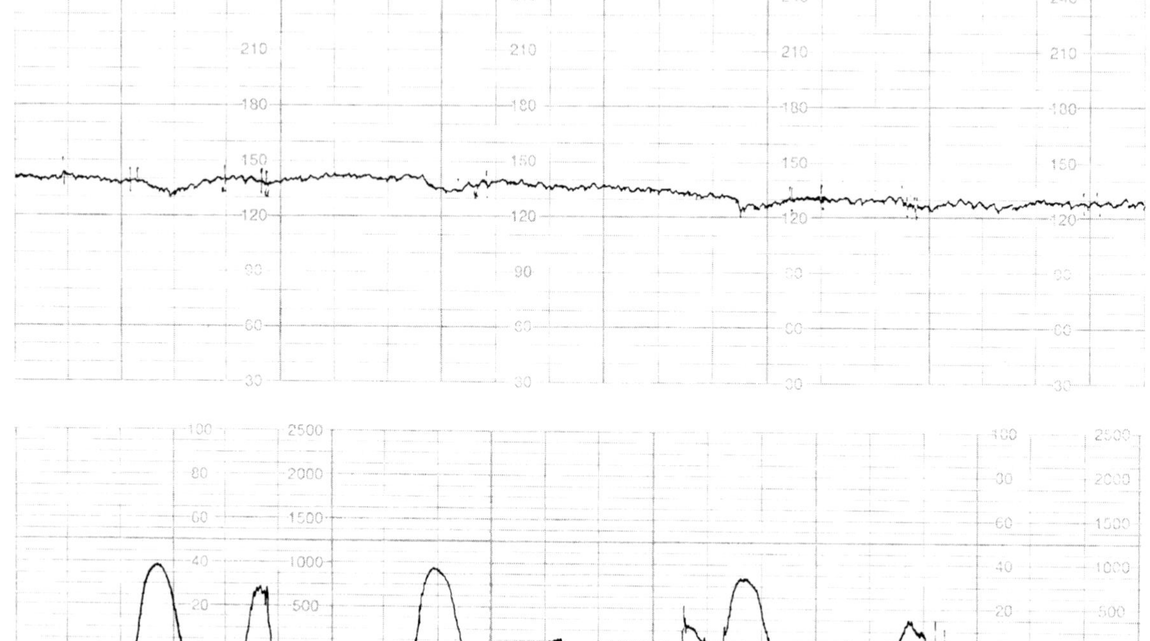

CTG at 16.00 hours.

16.00 hours

CTG (Fig. 4.35, part 2).

CTG

1 What do you notice about the baseline?
2 What do you notice about the baseline variability?
3 What periodic changes, if any, are present?
4 What do you notice about the uterine activity?
5 Would you categorise the CTG as normal/suspicious/ pathological?
6 What is the most probable cause of fetal heart rate abnormality shown on this trace?
7 What treatment and/or intervention would you consider necessary for this fetal heart rate pattern?

NOTES

1

2

3

4

5

6

7

ANALYSIS

1 Baseline 140–150 bpm **Reassuring**
2 Less than 5 beats **Non-reassuring**
3 Possibly very shallow late decelerations **Abnormal**
4 Contracting irregularly, varying in strength; inadequately monitored.
5 There is one abnormal and one non-reassuring feature: the CTG is classified as pathological.
6 Administration of pethidine 15 minutes prior to portion of CTG could explain the reduction in variability; however, in view of previous CTG and fresh meconium-stained liquor, fetal compromise must be considered.
7 Fetal blood sampling is indicated.
If pattern persists, prepare for delivery.

OUTCOME

17.00 hours

Cervical os 5 cm dilated.
Fetal blood sampling performed: pH 7.20, base deficit 10 mmol/l, warrants immediate delivery.
Caesarean section performed.
Live girl.
Apgar score 9/1 9/5.
Birthweight 4.560 kg.
Cord around neck × 1 and around leg × 2.
No cord blood sample available.

Miscellaneous

SECTION **10**

Fig. 4.36

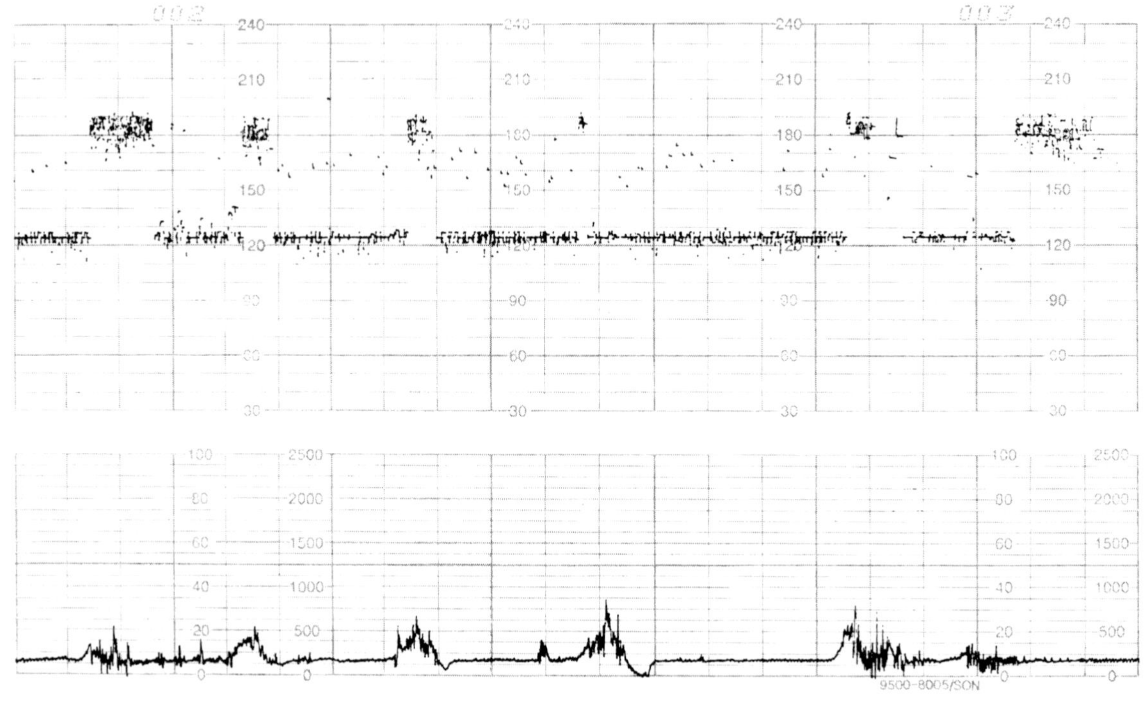

HISTORY

24-year-old gravida 2, para 1.

Past history

Nil relevant.

Antenatal period

Normal.
Admitted at 40 weeks with spontaneous rupture of membranes and contractions.

Labour

10.30 hours

Cervical os 5 cm dilated.
Clear liquor draining.
Fetal scalp electrode applied.
Contractions monitored externally.
Transcutaneous nerve stimulation for analgesia.
CTG (Fig. 4.36).

CTG

1. What do you notice about the baseline?
2. What do you notice about the baseline variability?
3. What periodic changes, if any, are present?
4. What do you notice about the uterine activity?
5. Would you categorise the CTG as normal/suspicious/pathological?
6. What is the most probable cause of fetal heart rate abnormality shown on this trace?
7. What treatment and/or intervention would you consider necessary for this fetal heart rate pattern?

NOTES

1

2

3

4

5

6

7

ANALYSIS

Impossible to interpret this CTG, owing to electrical interference from transcutaneous nerve stimulation.
Fetal heart should be auscultated and rate written on CTG.
The woman is in a low-risk category so continuous CTG should not be recommended unless it is her choice. A CTG with poor recording is of no value and should be discontinued.

OUTCOME

12.30 hours

Second stage of labour diagnosed.

12.50 hours

Spontaneous vertex delivery.
Live girl.
Apgar score 9/1 9/5.
Birthweight 3.560 kg.

Fig. 4.37

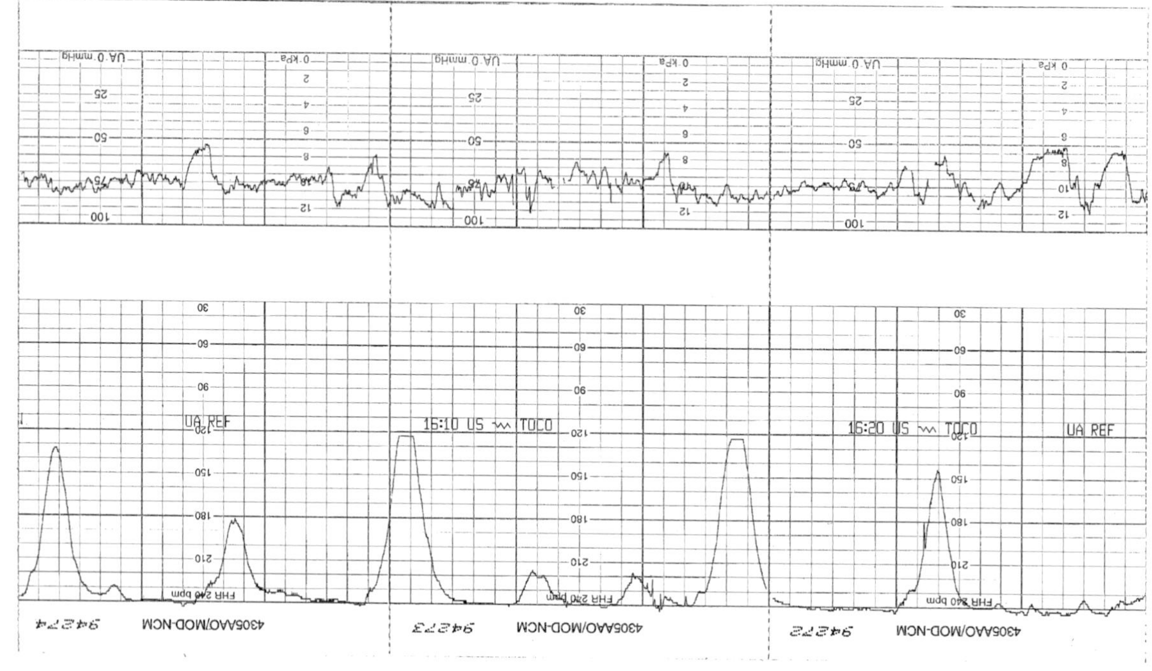

HISTORY

27-year-old gravida 3, para 2.

Past history

Nil relevant.

Antenatal period

Urinary tract infection treated at 24 weeks' gestation.
Normal progress.
Admitted at 41 weeks' gestation in spontaneous labour.

Labour

13.30 hours

Cervical os 5 cm dilated, membranes intact.
Initial CTG normal.

15.50 hours

CTG recommenced, external recordings (Fig. 4.37).

CTG

1. What do you notice about the baseline?
2. What do you notice about the baseline variability?
3. What periodic changes, if any, are present?
4. What do you notice about the uterine activity?
5. Would you categorise the CTG as normal/suspicious/pathological?
6. What is the most probable cause of fetal heart rate abnormality shown on this trace?
7. What treatment and/or intervention would you consider necessary for this fetal heart rate pattern?

NOTES

1

2

3

4

5

6

7

ANALYSIS

1 Baseline, unable to interpret.
2 Variability, probably within normal limits.
3 Accelerations present, no decelerations.
4 Contracting 3 in 10 minutes, varying in strength.
5 Probably normal CTG: paper has been loaded into machine upside-down. Despite this the CTG is recorded as being satisfactory in the case notes on two occasions.
6 Change paper.

OUTCOME

Paper rectified after 1 hour.
Progressed to normal birth 3 hours later.
Live girl.
Apgar score 9/1 9/5.
Birthweight 3.380 kg.

DISCUSSION

Although on first glance this CTG appears normal it is not apparent that the paper is upside down until closer inspection. The CTG had been interpreted and documented as normal on a number of occasions until the error was identified and rectified.

This calls into question the experience of the practitioners who interpreted the CTG. If a systematic approach is used to describe the features this should have been identified immediately.

In this case the fetal heart rate was normal; however if there had been abnormalities it would have been very difficult to categorise them clearly and the potential for serious omissions is great.

It is a reminder that vigilance is necessary at all times when using technology and we should not be complacent. We should remember that something as simple as reloading paper into the monitor can still be done wrongly.

Fig. 4.38, Part 1

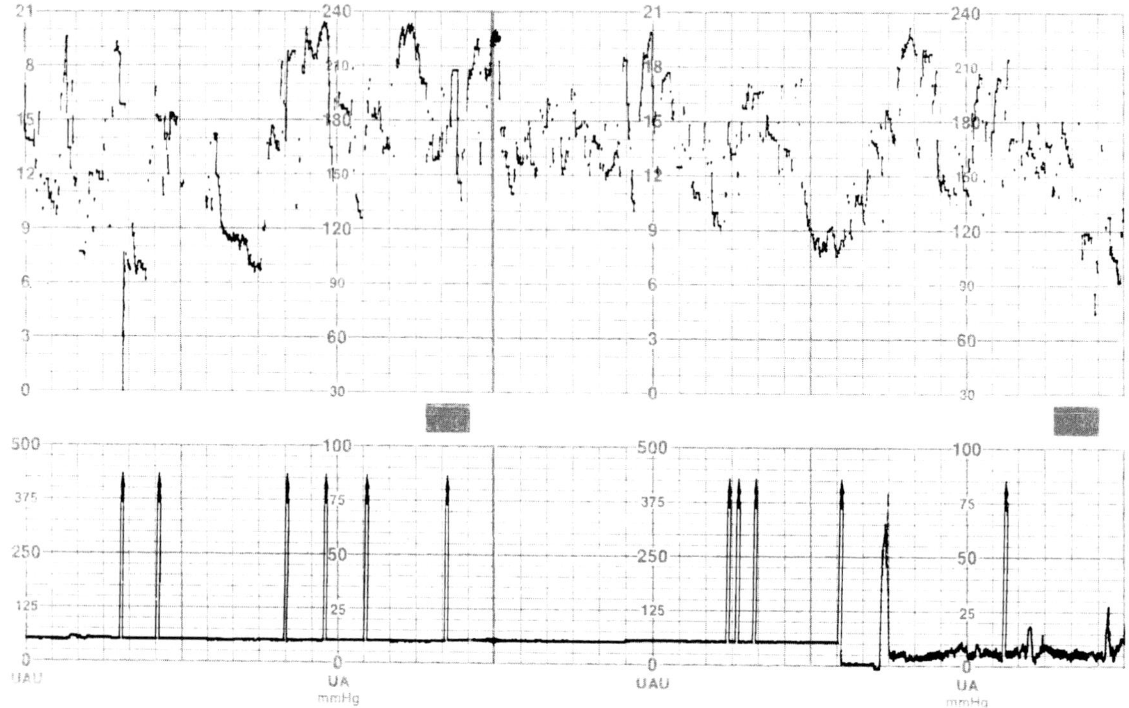

HISTORY

30-year-old gravida 1, para 0.

Past history

Nil relevant.

Antenatal period

Admitted at 31 weeks with pregnancy-induced hypertension.
Admission CTG normal.
Blood pressure stabilised.
32 weeks.
Ultrasound scan shows good growth and normal liquor volume.
Routine CTG 2 days later (Fig. 4.38, part 1).

CTG

1. What do you notice about the baseline?
2. What do you notice about the baseline variability?
3. What periodic changes, if any, are present?
4. What do you notice about the uterine activity?
5. Would you categorise the CTG as normal/suspicious/pathological?
6. What is the most probable cause of fetal heart rate abnormality shown on this trace?
7. What treatment and/or intervention would you consider necessary for this fetal heart rate pattern?

NOTES

1

2

3

4

5

6

7

ANALYSIS

Impossible to interpret this CTG. The baseline could be below 120 bpm or above 180 bpm. In the few areas where it is possible to measure, the variability appears to be more than 5 beats. Depending on where the baseline is placed, there are either decelerations or accelerations present. It is not safe to base actions on this CTG; however further investigation is warranted.

Fetal heart sounded irregular. Repeat CTG – similar pattern.

Case 38 continued over page.

Case 38 continued

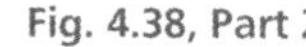

Fig. 4.38, Part 2

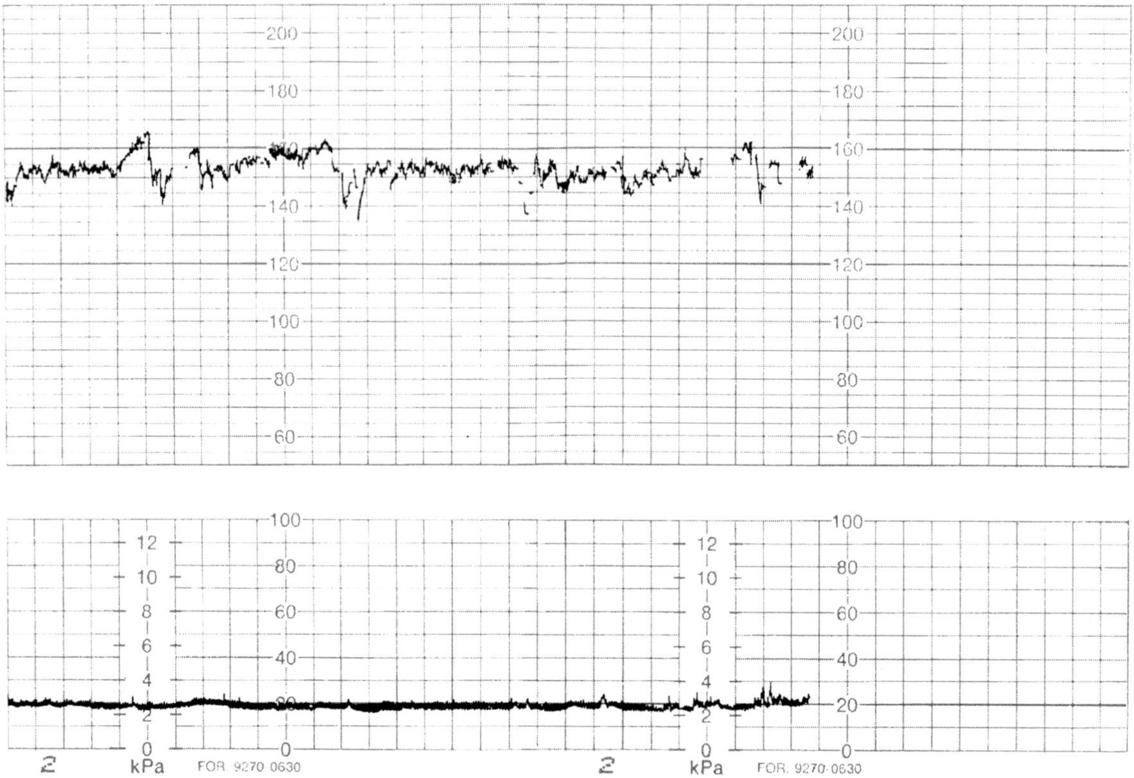

OUTCOME

Ultrasound scan performed.
Structurally normal heart – atrial flutter diagnosed.
Cardiology opinion sought.
Mother digitalised.
Following day – ultrasound scan shows fetal heart in normal sinus rhythm.
CTG repeated 2 days later (Fig 4.38, part 2).
35 weeks.
Blood pressure unstable.
Caesarean section performed.
Live girl.
Apgar score 4/1 9/5.
Birthweight 1.810 kg.
Baby discharged at 3 weeks old – no problems.

Fig. 4.39

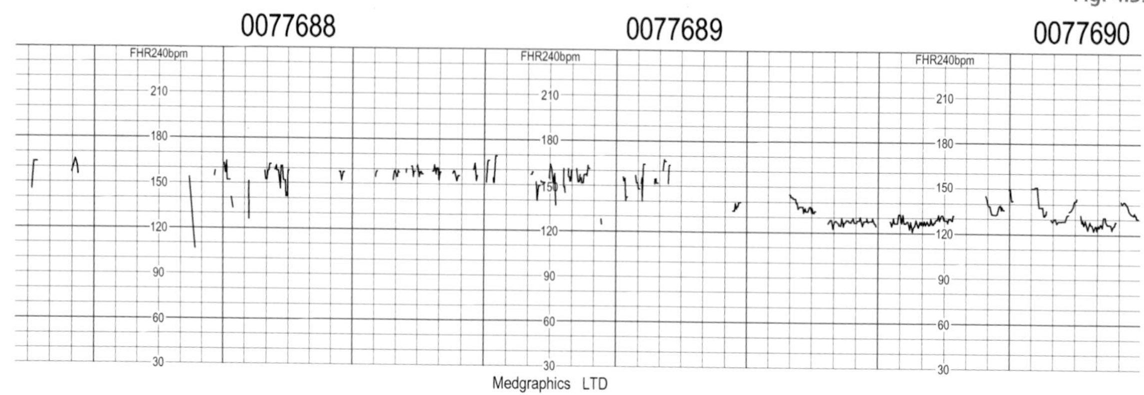

HISTORY

29-year-old gravida 3, para 2.

Past history

Nil of note.

Antenatal period

Normal.
Admitted in spontaneous labour at 40 weeks' gestation.

Labour

06.30 hours

Vaginal assessment revealed the cervix to be thin and well applied to presenting part; the cervical os was 4 cm dilated. No analgesia was in use.
CTG (Fig. 4.39).

CTG

1 What do you notice about the baseline?
2 What do you notice about the baseline variability?
3 What periodic changes, if any, are present?
4 What do you notice about the uterine activity?
5 Would you categorise the CTG as normal/suspicious/pathological?
6 What is the most probable cause of fetal heart rate abnormality shown on this trace?
7 What treatment and/or intervention would you consider necessary for this fetal heart rate pattern?

NOTES

1

2

3

4

5

6

7

ANALYSIS

1 Baseline difficult to decide due to poor contact, possibly 130 bpm.
2 Variability: again poor contact makes this difficult, possibly 5 beats.
3 Possibly no decelerations with some acceleration.
4 Contractions not monitored.
5 This could be a normal CTG, but the quality is too poor to be certain.
6 Unable to identify abnormalities or causes.
7 Ensure good contact, monitor contractions. This woman was deemed to be low risk for labour; the reason for the CTG should be questioned. Intermittent auscultation should be offered as the preferred method of monitoring the fetal heart rate in labour. If the woman chooses to have continuous monitoring then the risks and benefits as explained to her must be documented in the case notes and her informed consent gained.

OUTCOME

Labour progressed well and a live boy was born 2 hours later.
Apgar score 9/1 9/5.
Birthweight 3.860 kg.

DISCUSSION

In fact intermittent auscultation had been used throughout this labour.

The CTG monitor had been used when auscultating the fetal heart and recorded each time it was listened to; note the times preprinted on the paper. This gives the impression of a continuous CTG. When performing intermittent auscultation the fetal heart rate must be counted for a full minute, with a Pinard stethoscope or hand-held Doppler, not a CTG transducer. There should be no recording as this may lead to someone wrongly interpreting the data and potentially initiating unnecessary interventions.

Fig. 4.40, Part 1

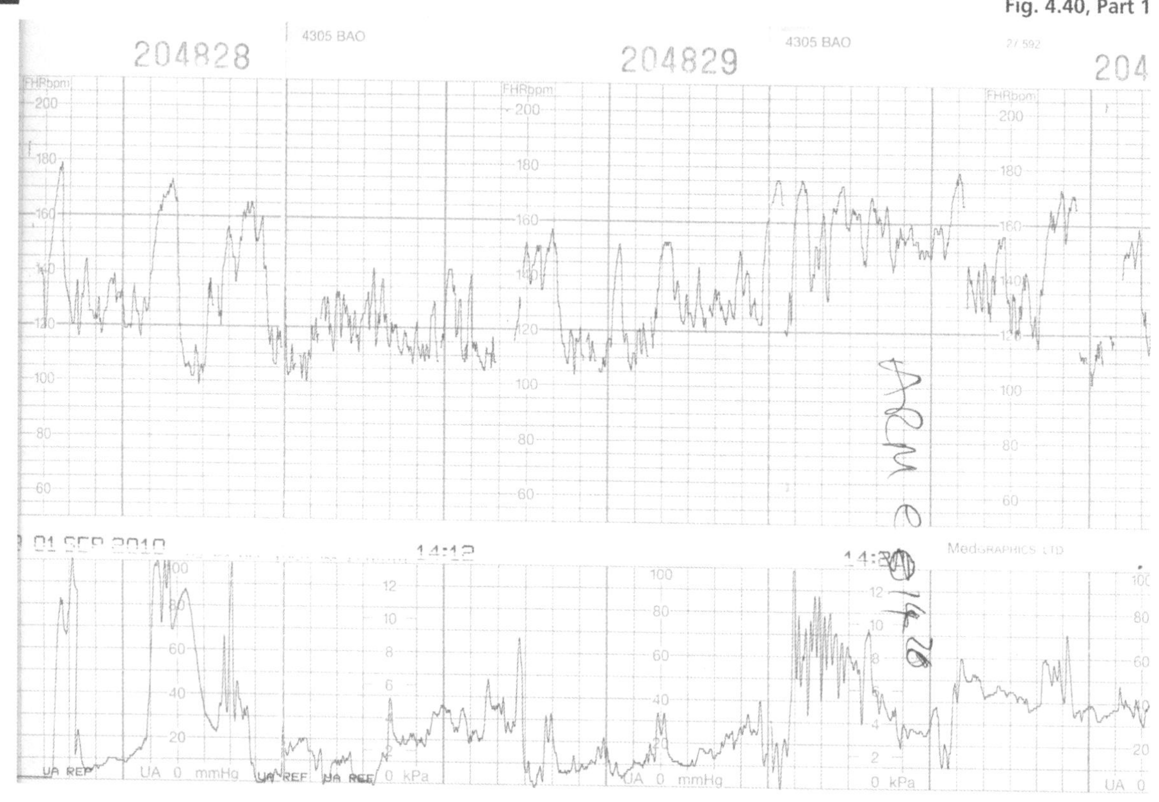

HISTORY

33-year-old gravida 2, para 1.

Past history

Asthmatic.

Antenatal period

Well, no problems identified. Low risk, midwifery-led care.
Baby on 50th centile on serial symphysiofundal height measurements.

Labour

Admitted at 41 weeks in spontaneous labour. Gave history of fresh bleeding per vaginam, approximately 2 tablespoons. Not a show, no evidence of rupture of membranes. Cervical os 3 cm dilated. Fetal heart rate auscultated at 120 bpm, fetal movements normal, currently active.
CTG commenced in view of bleeding. Maternal observations of pulse, temperature, blood pressure and respiration rate are within normal limits.
CTG (Fig. 4.40, Part 1).

CTG

1. What do you notice about the baseline?
2. What do you notice about the baseline variability?
3. What periodic changes, if any, are present?
4. What do you notice about the uterine activity?
5. Would you categorise the CTG as normal/suspicious/pathological?
6. What is the most probable cause of fetal heart rate abnormality shown on this trace?
7. What treatment and/or intervention would you consider necessary for this fetal heart rate pattern?

NOTES

1

2

3

4

5

6

7

ANALYSIS

1 Baseline 110–120 bpm **Reassuring**
2 Variability 5–10 beats **Reassuring**
3 Accelerations present **Reassuring**
No decelerations **Reassuring**
4 Contracting 2:10 minutes.
5 All features are reassuring: the CTG is classified as normal.
6 No abnormalities.
7 Continue CTG in view of history of bleeding.

OUTCOME

In view of vaginal bleeding artificial rupture of the membranes was performed. Clear liquor was draining, although the colour of the liquor and cervical dilatation are not documented on the CTG.
10 minutes following artificial rupture of the membranes, CTG.
CTG (Fig. 4.40, Part 2).

Case 40 continued over page.

Case 40 continued

Fig. 4.40, Part 2

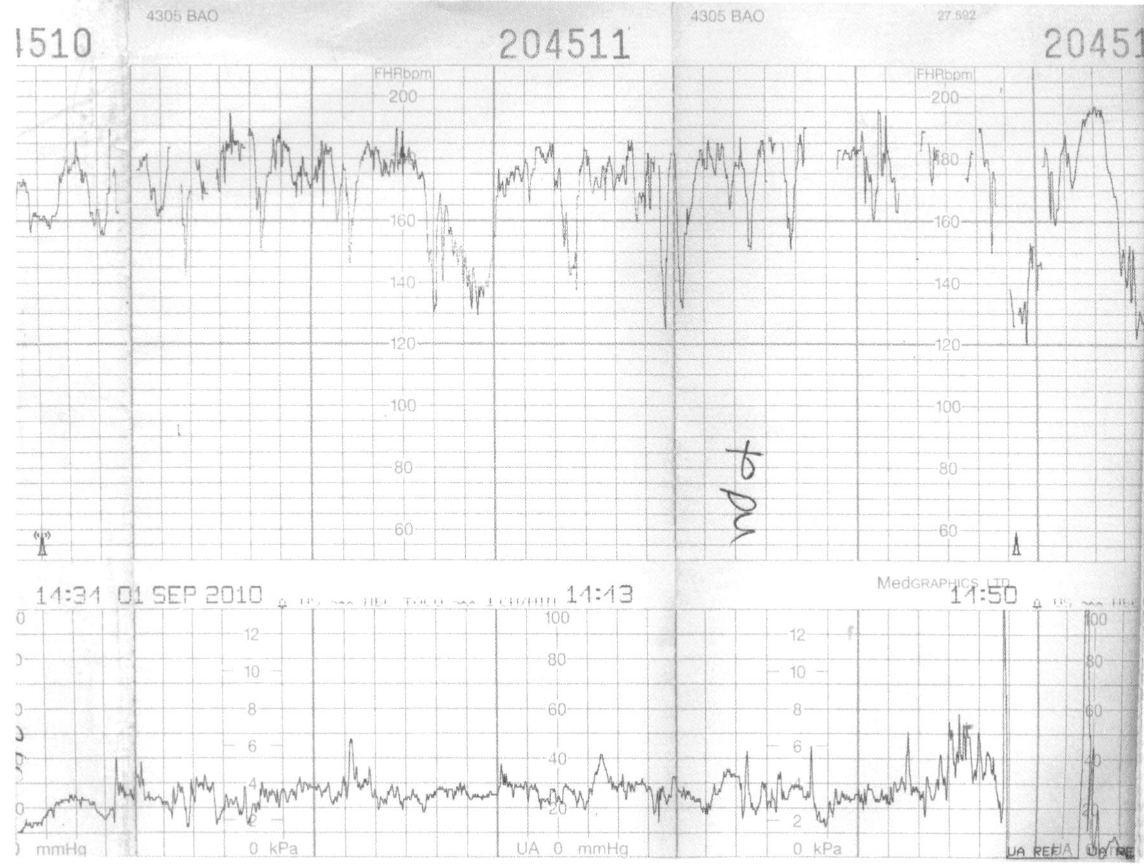

CTG

1 What do you notice about the baseline?
2 What do you notice about the baseline variability?
3 What periodic changes, if any, are present?
4 What do you notice about the uterine activity?
5 Would you categorise the CTG as normal/suspicious/pathological?
6 What is the most probable cause of fetal heart rate abnormality shown on this trace?
7 What treatment and/or intervention would you consider necessary for this fetal heart rate pattern?

NOTES

1

2

3

4

5

6

7

ANALYSIS

1	Baseline 180 bpm	**Non-reassuring**
2	Variability 5–10 beats	**Reassuring**
3	Atypical variable decelerations. No accelerations	**Abnormal**

4 Contractions not adequately monitored.

5 There is one non-reassuring and one abnormal feature: the CTG is classified as pathological.

6 The decelerations are caused by cord compression; as they are atypical they are suggestive of developing hypoxia. Determining a cause for the increase in baseline heart rate is not so easy. Potentially maternal pyrexia has developed; the temperature on admission was normal. The variability is normal, which does not suggest fetal compromise. There has been vaginal bleeding so there is a possibility that this has been underestimated and has been sufficient to cause symptoms in the woman such as a tachycardia with a resultant fetal heart rate tachycardia. Is this a true fetal heart rate tachycardia or could it be reactivity to fetal movements?

7 Record maternal observations to exclude pyrexia and tachycardia.
Observe for further vaginal blood loss.
Ask the woman if the baby is currently active.
Consider fetal blood sampling.

OUTCOME

No further blood loss was observed. Maternal observations were not performed. Medical opinion was sought regarding fetal blood sampling. 5 minutes later CTG (Fig. 4.40, Part 3).

Case 40 continued over page.

Case 40 continued

Fig. 4.40, Part 3

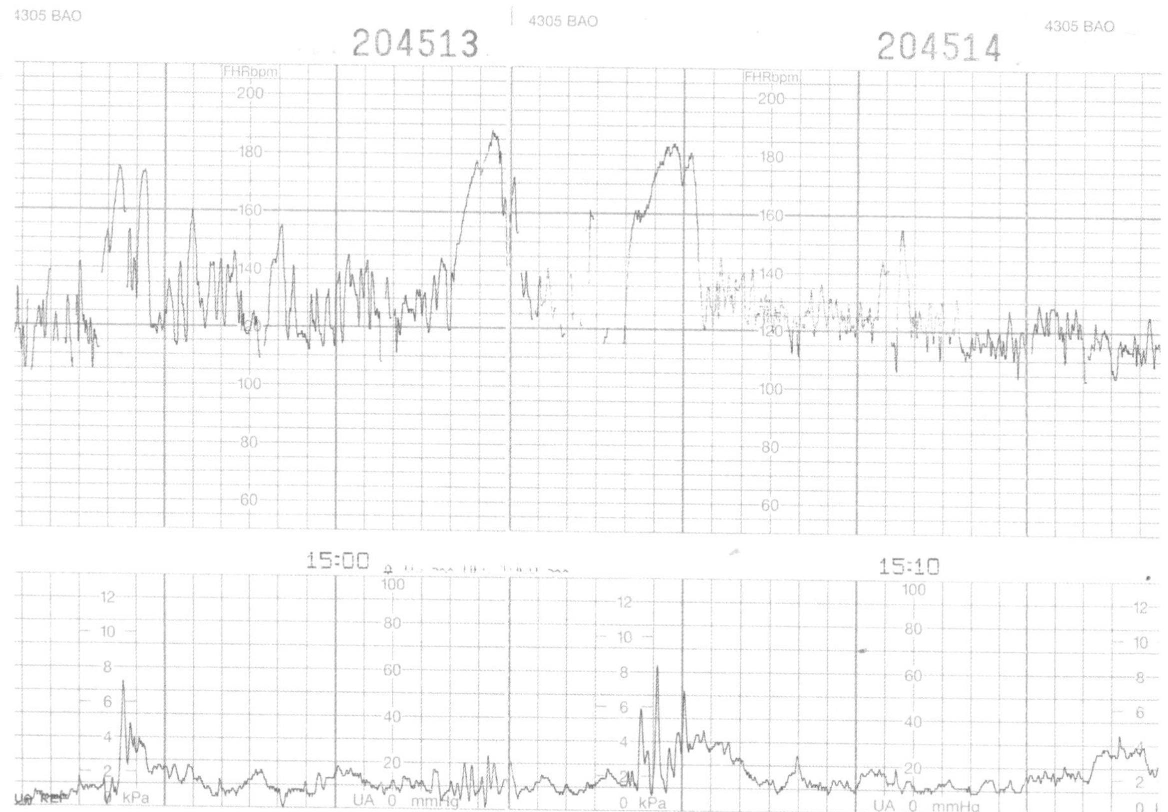

CTG

1 What do you notice about the baseline?
2 What do you notice about the baseline variability?
3 What periodic changes, if any, are present?
4 What do you notice about the uterine activity?
5 Would you categorise the CTG as normal/suspicious/pathological?
6 What is the most probable cause of fetal heart rate abnormality shown on this trace?
7 What treatment and/or intervention would you consider necessary for this fetal heart rate pattern?

NOTES

1

2

3

4

5

6

7

ANALYSIS

1	Baseline 110–120 bpm	Reassuring
2	Variability 5–10 beats	Reassuring
3	Accelerations present	Reassuring
	No decelerations	Reassuring
4	Contracting 2:10 minutes, not monitored adequately.	
5	All features are reassuring: the CTG is classified as normal.	
6	No abnormalities.	
7	Continue CTG in view of history of bleeding.	

DISCUSSION

The pattern on the previous portion of CTG probably occurred as a result of fetal activity. There was documentation in the labour record confirming that the baby was active at this time, although there was no documentation on the CTG. Asking the woman if the baby is active at the time of the CTG is beneficial and can be reassuring for the professional, reducing anxiety for both the clinician and the woman and partner. This also demonstrates the importance of looking at the entire CTG rather than a small portion, as well as the documentation in the records. Communication between the midwife and obstetrician is vital to establish appropriate management. Unnecessary interventions can be made when jumping to conclusions without full information and exploration of the possible causes of a CTG abnormality, particularly when a deviation from normal has been identified, such as vaginal bleeding.

OUTCOME

Labour progressed well. Normal birth occurred 3 hours after the last portion of CTG. Live girl, Apgar score 9/1 9/5, birthweight 3.640 kg.
No cord blood samples were obtained.

Fig. 4.41

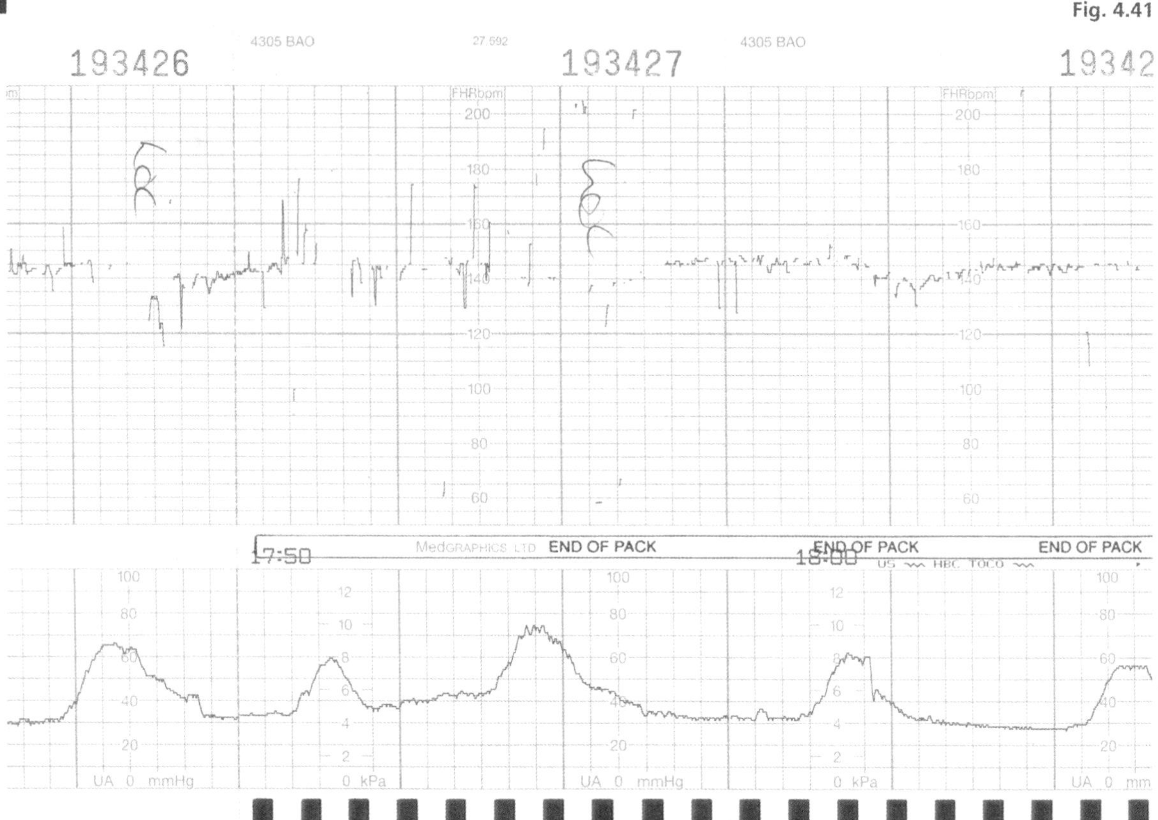

HISTORY

25-year-old gravida 2, para 0 + 1.

Past history

No problems, normally fit and well.

Antenatal period

Well until 35 weeks. Growth noted to be tailing off, ultrasound scan confirmed estimated weight just above 10th centile. 37 weeks: admitted with reduced fetal movements, liquor volume reduced with absent end diastolic flow. Labour induced with Propess.

Labour

Contractions commenced 2 hours after administration of Propess. Vaginal examination not performed, CTG commenced.
CTG (Fig. 4.41).

CTG

1 What do you notice about the baseline?
2 What do you notice about the baseline variability?
3 What periodic changes, if any, are present?
4 What do you notice about the uterine activity?
5 Would you categorise the CTG as normal/suspicious/pathological?
6 What is the most probable cause of fetal heart rate abnormality shown on this trace?
7 What treatment and/or intervention would you consider necessary for this fetal heart rate pattern?

NOTES

1

2

3

4

5

6

7

ANALYSIS

1 Baseline difficult to assess with accuracy due to poor quality. Appears to be around 140 bpm — **Reassuring**
2 Again, not easy to determine, appears less than 5 beats — **Non-reassuring**
3 No accelerations present
Possibly some late decelerations, see around 18.00 hours — **Abnormal**
4 Contracting 3:10 minutes.
5 There is one non-reassuring and one abnormal feature, although it is difficult to be certain due to the poor quality of CTG: CTG would be classified as pathological.
6 A decrease in variability along with late decelerations are indicative of fetal hypoxia. The history of reduced fetal movements, absent end diastolic flow and tailing off of growth are signs of poor placental function which would lead to a fetus with reduced reserves, less able to cope with the stress of labour.
7 Fetal blood sample should be considered if the cervical dilatation is optimal. The quality of the recording must be improved. It is not possible to be certain about the analysis of this CTG. In this case, where there is a baby at risk of developing CTG abnormalities in labour, it is vital that the recording is of good quality to ensure that abnormalities are clearly shown and appropriate management initiated. Where contact is lost it is not sufficient to document 'LOC' (loss of contact). The fetal heart rate must be auscultated and the rate written on the CTG. Maternal pulse should also be recorded.

OUTCOME

The CTG was continued. One hour later, variable decelerations apparent on CTG. Cervical dilatation not sufficient to allow fetal blood sampling, therefore caesarean section performed.
Baby boy, Apgar score 9/1 9/5, birthweight 2.890 kg.

Cord blood analysis results were within normal limits.

	pH	Base deficit (mmol/l)
UA	7.259	2
UV	7.303	4.1

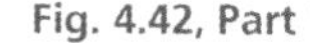

Fig. 4.42, Part 1

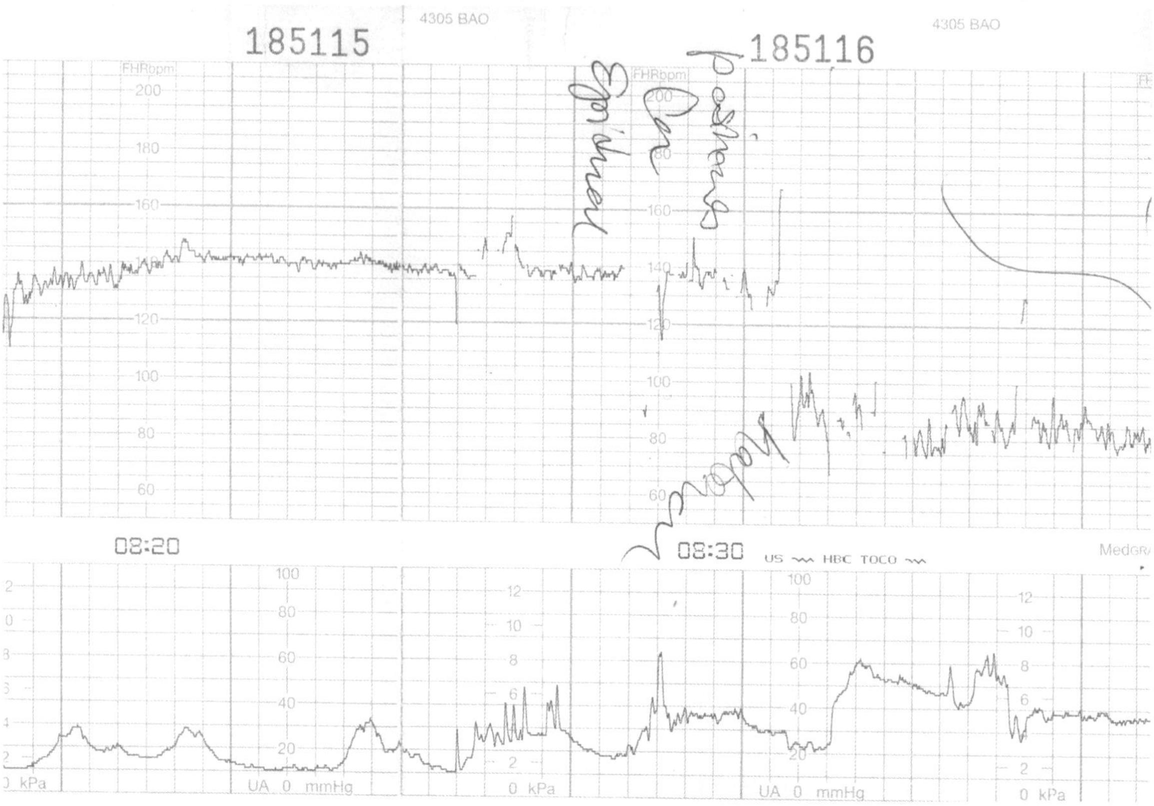

HISTORY

28-year-old gravida 2, para 1.

Past history

No problems, normally fit and well.

Antenatal period

Well throughout, growth just below 90th centile on serial symphysiofundal height measurements. Low risk, midwifery-led care.

Labour

Admitted to midwifery-led birth centre in spontaneous labour at 40 weeks' gestation. Fetal heart auscultated at 136 bpm. Mobilising, no analgesia. Vaginal assessment not performed. Two hours later requesting epidural analgesia. Cervical dilatation 5 cm. Transferred to labour ward for epidural.
On arrival, CTG commenced, despite still being in a low-risk category.
CTG (Fig. 4.42, Part 1).

CTG

1 What do you notice about the baseline?
2 What do you notice about the baseline variability?
3 What periodic changes, if any, are present?
4 What do you notice about the uterine activity?
5 Would you categorise the CTG as normal/suspicious/pathological?
6 What is the most probable cause of fetal heart rate abnormality shown on this trace?
7 What treatment and/or intervention would you consider necessary for this fetal heart rate pattern?

NOTES

1

2

3

4

5

6

7

ANALYSIS

1 Baseline 140 bpm — **Reassuring**
2 Variability 5 beats — **Reassuring**
3 Accelerations present — **Reassuring**
No decelerations — **Reassuring**
4 Contracting 3:10 minutes, although not monitored adequately.
5 All features are reassuring, CTG is classified as normal.
6 Once positioned for epidural insertion the fetal heart rate appears to drop to a baseline of 80–90 bpm. This is documented on the CTG as 'maternal pulse'. We do not know the position the woman is in and there is potential to interpret this as a prolonged deceleration.
7 The exact position the woman has adopted should be written on the CTG. In addition it is important to write in the maternal pulse rate to confirm that it is maternal pulse recording. The fetal heart rate should also be auscultated and the rate written on the CTG. If it is difficult to maintain adequate contact and recording of the fetal heart rate, it may be necessary to discontinue the CTG, auscultate the fetal heart rate and recommence the CTG after the insertion of the epidural.

OUTCOME

Epidural insertion continued.
CTG (Fig. 4.42, Part 2).

Case 42 continued over page.

Case 42 continued

Fig. 4.42, Part 2

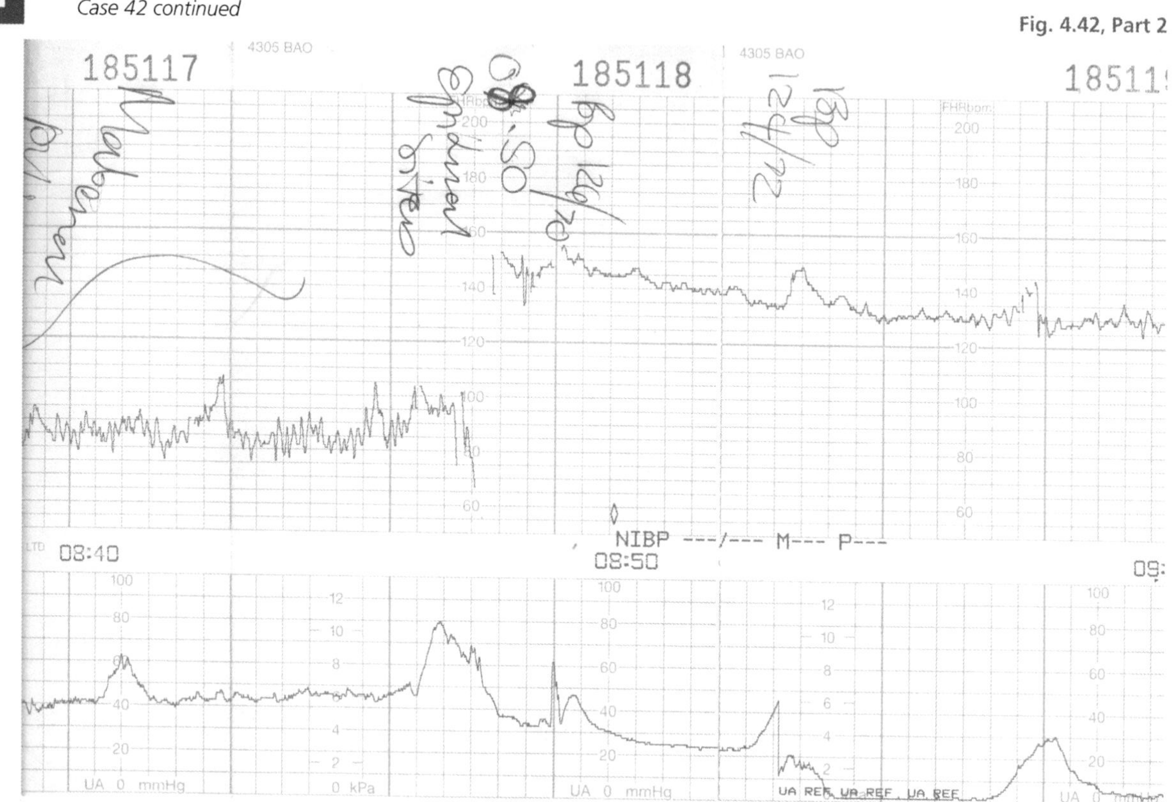

CTG

1 What do you notice about the baseline?
2 What do you notice about the baseline variability?
3 What periodic changes, if any, are present?
4 What do you notice about the uterine activity?
5 Would you categorise the CTG as normal/suspicious/pathological?
6 What is the most probable cause of fetal heart rate abnormality shown on this trace?
7 What treatment and/or intervention would you consider necessary for this fetal heart rate pattern?

NOTES

1

2

3

4

5

6

7

ANALYSIS

1 Baseline 140 bpm **Reassuring**
2 Variability 5 beats **Reassuring**
3 Accelerations present **Reassuring**
No decelerations **Reassuring**
4 Contracting 3:10 minutes, although not monitored adequately.
5 All features are reassuring, CTG is classified as normal.
6 Although it is not documented on the CTG it is assumed that the woman changes position after the insertion of the epidural and contact with the fetal heart is resumed. Blood pressure recordings are documented, although the amount and strength of drug given via the epidural are not.
7 The CTG demonstrates the importance of documenting the maternal pulse rate in beats rather than writing 'maternal pulse' as it could be argued at a later date that this was in fact the fetal heart rate.

OUTCOME

Second stage of labour was diagnosed 2 hours 45 minutes later. The CTG remained in progress throughout labour, no abnormalities detected.
Normal birth, baby girl, Apgar score 8/1 9/5, birthweight 3180 kg.
No cord blood sample obtained.

DISCUSSION

There are a few issues worthy of discussion. Firstly, why was this CTG commenced? The woman was transferred to the labour ward for epidural analgesia. This would not place her in a high-risk category. A CTG should be performed for 20–30 minutes after the administration of a bolus dose of analgesia via the epidural cannula then discontinued if normal.

It is important to write the rate of the maternal pulse rather than just 'maternal pulse' to confirm that it has been investigated. It it is also advisable to auscultate the fetal heart rate and document the rate on the CTG.

It is interesting to note that the pattern of the maternal pulse rate is virtually indistinguishable from a fetal heart rate recording on a CTG, apart from the actual rate. If the maternal pulse was raised this would appear to be a fetal heart. It highlights how, in the absence of a fetal heart rate when the CTG picks up maternal pulse, it is possible to be convinced that the fetal heart rate is present.

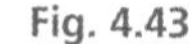

Fig. 4.43

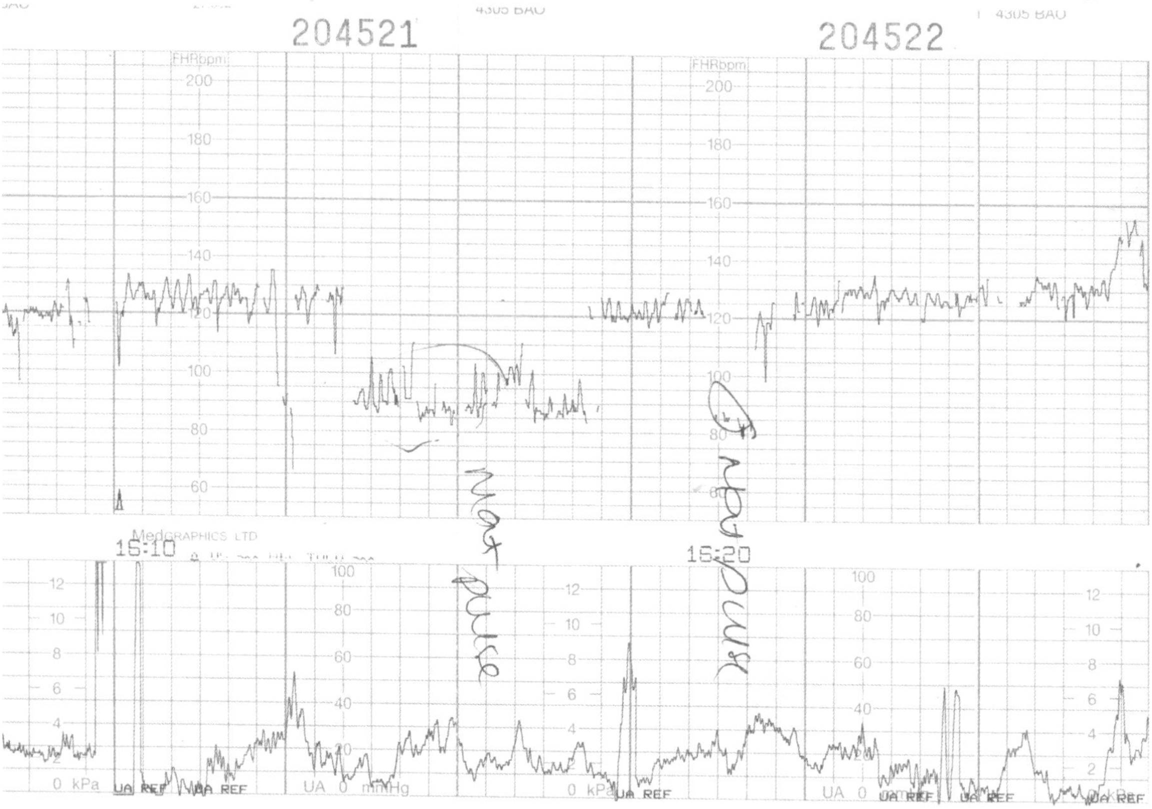

HISTORY

20-year-old gravida 2, para 1.

Past history

Previous normal birth.
Type 1 diabetes, insulin-dependent.

Antenatal period

Diabetes well controlled throughout.

Labour

Admitted at 38 weeks' gestation in spontaneous labour.
Contracting 3:10. Cervical os 6 cm dilated.
CTG (Fig. 4.43).

CTG

1 What do you notice about the baseline?
2 What do you notice about the baseline variability?
3 What periodic changes, if any, are present?
4 What do you notice about the uterine activity?
5 Would you categorise the CTG as normal/suspicious/pathological?
6 What is the most probable cause of fetal heart rate abnormality shown on this trace?
7 What treatment and/or intervention would you consider necessary for this fetal heart rate pattern?

NOTES

1

2

3

4

5

6

7

ANALYSIS

1 Baseline 120–130 bpm **Reassuring**
2 Variability 5–10 beats **Reassuring**
3 Accelerations present **Reassuring**
No decelerations **Reassuring**
4 Contracting 3:10 minutes, although not monitored adequately.
5 All features are reassuring, CTG is classified as normal.
6 There are no abnormalities identified.
7 There is a period of 4 minutes when the fetal heart rate appears to drop to 90 bpm and a further 1-minute portion soon afterwards. Both have been circled and 'maternal pulse' written on the CTG. The actual maternal pulse rate should be written on the CTG along with the auscultated fetal heart rate to confirm that this is really maternal pulse and not a decelerative episode. This is a high-risk pregnancy and monitoring must be accurate.

OUTCOME

Progress in labour was good, normal birth 2 hours after CTG.
Live boy, Apgar score 9/1 9/5, birthweight 4.100 kg.
Cord blood samples not available.

DISCUSSION

The areas where maternal pulse have been recorded on the CTG have been circled. This is not approprate and adds nothing to the interpretation of the CTG. There is a potential for this to obliterate the printout, making analysis more difficult. The same applies when decelerations occur and the nadir is circled or underlined. It is sufficient to make a note in the labour record that the CTG has been analysed and place a signature or initials upon the CTG with the category of CTG, well away from the printout to avoid covering the data.

REFERENCE

National Collborating Centre for Women's and Children's Health (NCCWCH). (2007) *Intrapartum Care. Care of healthy women and their babies during childbirth*. London: RCOG Press. (Clinical Guideline).

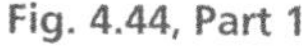
Fig. 4.44, Part 1

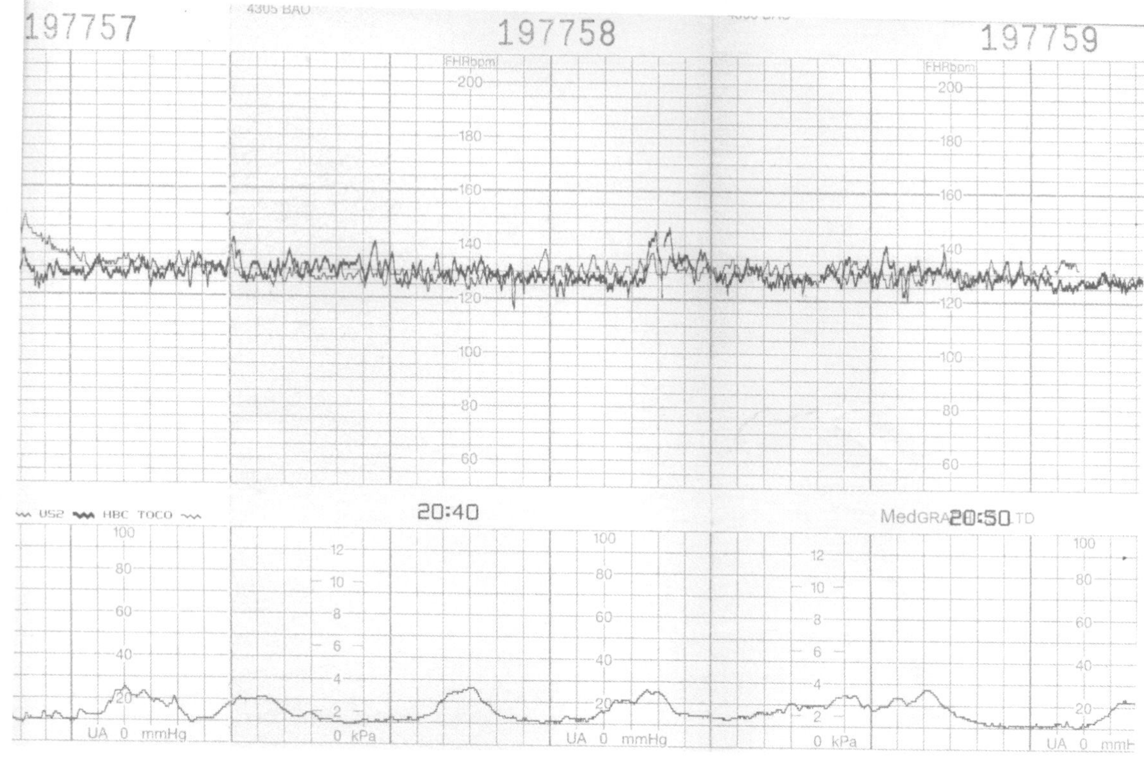

HISTORY

29-year-old gravida 4, para 3.

Past history

Two previous normal births.
No problems, normally fit and well.

Antenatal period

Twin pregnancy, dichorionic, diamniotic.
Well throughout, serial ultrasound scans, both twins growing along the 50th centile.
Admitted at 35 weeks' gestation with contractions. Settled and returned home.

Labour

Readmitted at 36 + 4 weeks in active labour. Membranes ruptures, clear liquor draining, cervical os 5 cm dilated. Both twins cephalic presentation. Fetal scalp electrode applied to twin 1.
CTG (Fig. 4.44, Part 1).

CTG

1. What do you notice about the baseline?
2. What do you notice about the baseline variability?
3. What periodic changes, if any, are present?
4. What do you notice about the uterine activity?
5. Would you categorise the CTG as normal/suspicious/pathological?
6. What is the most probable cause of fetal heart rate abnormality shown on this trace?
7. What treatment and/or intervention would you consider necessary for this fetal heart rate pattern?

NOTES

1

2

3

4

5

6

7

ANALYSIS

Twin 1 (dark line)

1 Baseline 135 bpm **Reassuring**
2 Variability 5–10 beats **Reassuring**
3 Accelerations present **Reassuring**
No decelerations **Reassuring**

Twin 2 (faint line)

Baseline 135 bpm **Reassuring**
Variability 5–10 beats **Reassuring**
Accelerations present **Reassuring**
No decelerations **Reassuring**

4 Contracting 3:10 minutes, although not monitored adequately.
5 All features are reassuring, CTG is classified as normal.
6 There are no abnormalities identified.
7 The CTG will continue as this is a high-risk pregnancy: twins at 36 + 4 weeks' gestation. The features on the CTG are similar for both twins and at times it may be difficult to interpret the CTG accurately if both lines are superimposed upon each other.
Modern CTG monitors allow the fetal heart rate recordings to be separated by 20 beats for a period of 10 minutes, enabling a more accurate interpretation.

Case 44 continued over page.

Case 44 continued

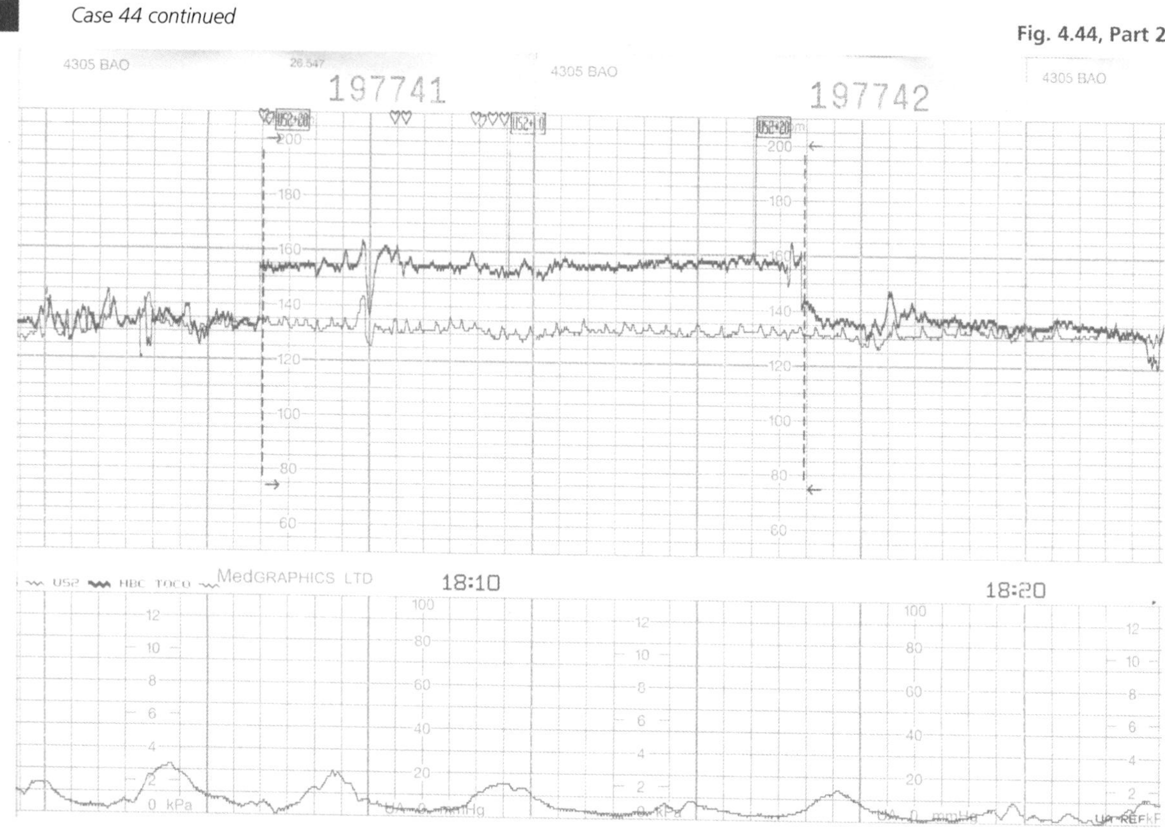

CTG (Fig. 4.44, Part 2)

Outcome

Labour progressed quickly, both twins had normal births.
Twin 1: girl. Apgar score 9/1 9/5, birthweight 3.050 kg.
Twin 2: boy. Apgar score 9/1 9/5, birthweight 3.120 kg.
Cord blood sample analysis results within normal limits.

	Twin 1		Twin 2	
	pH	Base deficit (mmol/l)	pH	Base deficit (mmol/l)
UA	7.280	8.8	7.264	6.3
UV	7.347	5.7	7.287	6

The pH measurements for twin 2 are lower than those of twin 1, which is be expected as twin 2 will have been subjected to a longer period of reduced oxygen transfer in the second stage of labour. The results are within normal limits and the base deficits are not suggestive of fetal hypoxia.

Good practice guide

PART 5

INTRODUCTION

Childbirth is a natural process for most women; however for some that process may be interrupted and deviates from normal, putting them and their unborn baby at risk. Midwives and obstetricians by the nature of their work become experienced in detecting when all is not well. The correct interpretation of the cardiotocograph (CTG), based on adequate knowledge of physiology, and the instigation of appropriate management are vital in ensuring that women and their babies are placed at as small risk as possible of harm due to negligence.

All professionals are responsible for ensuring that they remain updated in all aspects of clinical care, including the interpretation of CTGs, and together with their colleagues should make adequate provision for training and maintaining expertise within their employing trust.

It is hoped that this practical guide will assist practitioners to access information they may find beneficial and to highlight some areas of good practice that can be shared and disseminated.

DEVELOPING GUIDELINES

Government initiatives have prompted the development of evidence-based guidelines for assessing fetal well-being in labour (National Collborating Centre for Women's and Children's Health 2007) and clinical risk management standards for maternity services (NHS Litigation Authority 2009). However, each trust has responsibility to ensure that this guidance is incorporated into local guidelines and policies.

These guidelines should be developed by a multidisciplinary team and be evidence-based, clear, easily understood and accessible to all members of staff. It is essential that they are reviewed regularly and updated without delay if necessary. Ideally they should be accessible to all electronically. The practice of having many hard copies in clinical areas for reference can be problematic if changes to the guideline are made. There is the potential for both old and new copies to be in circulation, causing confusion as to current practice.

AUDIT

Audit of clinical practice is an essential component of the quality cycle. Standards and guidelines relating to assessment of fetal well-being in labour should be audited regularly to ensure that clinical practice continues to be in line with up-to-date evidence and that current practice equates with good clinical outcomes.

This audit can take many forms. Retrospective case note reviews to review record keeping, case reviews and root cause analysis investigations following untoward incidents, regular multidisciplinary discussion sessions and case presentations on labour wards are all beneficial and provide excellent learning opportunities for all professionals.

It is important that the findings and recommendations from completed audits must be disseminated to all staff. It is also important that any actions are followed through, with key staff members identified to instigate these.

COMMUNICATION

Regular, constructive, multidisciplinary discussions relating to the interpretation and management of CTG abnormalities have been advocated (NHS Litigation Authority 2009; National Collborating Centre for Women's and Children's Health 2007). Meetings should be well advertised, convenient for all groups of staff and conducted in a non-threatening manner. Attendance should be documented and form a part of the individual's personal development plan. Practitioners should also be encouraged to discuss the interpretation of CTGs when caring for women in labour. The senior midwife or obstetrician responsible for the department should ensure that this takes place at least once during the course of the shift.

The terminology used to describe the CTG must be consistent and used by all members of the labour ward team involved in the interpretation of CTGs. Pro formas to assist with the correct classification of CTGs have been developed (see Table 2.3).

TRAINING AND DEVELOPMENT

Ongoing training and development are paramount to maintain safe levels of practice relating to fetal heart rate monitoring. All practitioners should attend regular updates relating to CTG interpretation; however the providers must ensure that the updates are not repetitive, and are interesting and informative to encourage attendance. There is evidence to suggest that regular mandatory fetal heart rate monitoring education programmes have a positive effect upon perinatal outcomes (Westgate et al. 2007).

Providing this level of updating is a challenge. Birth rates are rising, midwives and obstetricians are busy providing increasingly high-risk care to women and the available time for training is reduced. Practitioners must have a degree of self-motivation to maintain their knowledge and skills; however not all education and training has to be delivered within a classroom setting.

'Issue of the week'-style notice boards can be utilised to highlight changes to guidelines, new evidence relating to fetal monitoring or CTG interpretation. Computer-based packages and training aids can be developed. E-mail is an excellent means of disseminating findings from audits and studies. Clinical practice-themed newsletters can also be generated and communicated on e-mail.

Training provision should also take into account the differing needs of professionals, unsocial working hours and ability to be released from clinical areas.

It may also be necessary to involve other groups of professionals such as the medical physics department within training, particularly when new equipment is introduced to the clinical area. Knowledge of how the CTG monitor works is as important as interpreting the data.

SUPERVISORS OF MIDWIVES

Supervisors of midwives are uniquely placed within the maternity services and should have a strong influence on clinical practice within their employing trusts. They should be represented on all guideline development groups and audit committees and be at the centre of developing and implementing practice changes. Supervisors meet with their supervisees a minimum of once per year. The discussions should include issues relating to fetal monitoring in labour, developments in clinical practice and the maintenance of clinical skills. In particular, with regard to the assessment of fetal well-being, use of the Pinard stethoscope should be encouraged. Drop-in sessions and workshops run by supervisors, in addition to the one-to-one meetings, allow for discussion and should be open to all staff.

PRACTICAL GUIDES

There are occasions when tools can be developed which prove beneficial to clinical practice. One such tool is highlighted here, currently in use at Birmingham Women's Health Care Foundation NHS Trust, and is replicated here with permission.

Fetal heart auscultation chart (Fig. 5.1)

This chart has been designed to be used during the second stage of labour in an attempt to make the documentation easier for the midwife. Accurate intermittent auscultation during the second stage of labour is not always easy, particularly if there is only one midwife present. By the time the woman is comfortable enough to have the Pinard or Doppler placed on her abdomen there is often another contraction commencing. It may be advisable to have two midwives present: one who can focus on supporting the woman, the other to auscultate the fetal heart rate.

The chart is designed to make recording easier by simply placing a dot to represent the fetal heart rtate rather than having to write it numerically after each auscultation. The chart is incorporated into the labour record following delivery.

RISK ASSESSMENT CHART

To minimise the risk of untoward occurrences/outcomes, the checklist in Table 5.1 has been compiled in relation to cardiotocography and should be used in conjunction with your employer's policies, protocols or guidelines and any rules, codes of practice and guidelines concerning the framework within which you practise as a doctor or midwife. For midwives, these will be those set out by the Nursing and Midwifery Council (NMC). For doctors they will be those of the employer.

Both groups must be familiar with any guidelines and/or protocols set out by an NHS trust or other place of work outside the NHS. This should also include advice and standards set by other recognised national bodies.

If the answer to any of the questions in Table 5.1 is 'no', then ask yourself 'What must I do about it?' Is it a matter for you, your colleagues, your supervisor of midwives, your manager?

It may be a useful tool to complete prior to a supervisory review meeting with your supervisor of midwives or practice performance review with your manager.

The NMC distributes the documents specified in Table 5.2 to all practitioners on the register. They are revised from time to time and it is the responsibility of each midwife to be familiar with their contents and refer to them as and when appropriate. If you do not have copies of any of the NMC documents on the list, then write to the NMC at: 23 Portland Place, London W1N 4JT.

Excellent communication is essential when developing good practice guides. This includes discussions with colleagues within the same unit and with those from other trusts. Sharing of information is vital and benchmarking practice and outcomes with other comparable units should be commonplace. Practitioners who have been involved in the planning and implementation of good-practice initiatives must be encouraged to write about their experiences and the benefits that can be demonstrated. Publishing of such work in professional journals will then provide the forum for dissemination of information and discussion.

Ultimately we practise within our professions in order to provide care for women and babies that will ensure they are as free from risk as possible. Happy, healthy families are the main aim; each individual practitioner has a duty to ensure that his/her practice does not hinder this.

Birmingham Women's Health Care NHS
NHS Trust

STICKY LABEL:

NAME:

REGISTRATION OR DATE OF BIRTH

(7) Version 2: Section 9: Labour Second Stage Fetal Heart Auscultation
(continue to complete the partogram documentation for all other observations)

DATE:...

NB: This is NOT intended to be used as a linear scale

To be auscultated after every contraction for a minimum of 1 minute (auscultation should be undertaken a minimum of every 5 minutes)

Fetal Heart Rate

190
180
170
160
150
140
130
120
110
100
90
80
70

Time commenced

TIME

Minimum of 1 contraction every five minutes

TIME	REASON FOR VARIANCE	SIGNATURE	CODE

Fig. 5.1 *Fetal heart auscultation chart.*

Table 5.1 Checklist of questions

	Yes	No
Are you confident and competent in the interpretation of the CTG?	❑	❑
Have you been trained and are you familiar with all the fetal monitoring equipment used in the clinical setting in which you work?	❑	❑
Are you aware of the facilities and personnel available for the repair and maintenance of equipment?	❑	❑
Are you satisfied with your knowledge of the research evidence, with regard to fetal monitoring, and do you base your practice upon this?	❑	❑
Are you comfortable in communicating any concerns regarding the interpretation of a CTG?	❑	❑
Do you obtain consent (informed) from women prior to commencing continuous fetal monitoring?	❑	❑
Do you attend regular multidisciplinary updating and training events in the interpretation of CTGs?	❑	❑
Is your record-keeping maintained to the highest standard? Is it clear, concise, legible and unambiguous?	❑	❑
When making records relating to a CTG, in the case notes, do you describe the baseline, variability, reactivity and presence or absence of any decelerations as opposed to writing 'normal' or 'satisfactory'?	❑	❑
Are you conversant with the current terminology (normal/suspicious/pathological) used to classify a CTG?	❑	❑
Is there a means of storing CTGs within the case notes that ensures that they do not get lost?	❑	❑

WEB ADDRESSES

There are a large number of easily accessible, useful websites. Some are listed below and most will have links to other sites. Many medical and midwifery journals are now available online, free of charge.

Association for Improvements in Maternity Services: <www.aims.org.uk>.

Confidential Enquiry into Maternal and Child Health: <www.cemach.org.uk>.

Table 5.2 Checklist of documents relating to practice

	Yes	No
Do you have a copy of the most up-to-date publications relevant to your practice, and are you familiar with their contents?	❑	❑
Midwives' Rules and Standards 2004	❑	❑
The Code, Standards of Conduct, Performance and Ethics for Nurses and Midwives 2008	❑	❑
Record Keeping: Guidance for Nurses and Midwives 2009	❑	❑
Are you familiar with all documents relating to areas of your practice?	❑	❑
Trust standards and guidelines	❑	❑
Royal College of Obstetricians and Gynaecologists advice and guidance	❑	❑
Nursing and Midwifery advice and guidance	❑	❑
The National Institute for Clinical Excellence guidelines	❑	❑
Clinical Negligence Scheme for Trusts standards	❑	❑
Local Supervising Authority for Midwives' standards	❑	❑

Department of Health: <www.doh.gov.uk>.

National Institute for Health and Clinical Excellence (NICE): <www.nice.org.uk>.

Nursing and Midwifery Council: <www.nmc-uk.org>.

Royal College of Obstetricians and Gynaecologists: <www.rcog.org.uk>.

REFERENCES

National Collborating Centre for Women's and Children's Health. (2007). *Intrapartum care. Care of healthy women and their babies during childbirth* (Clinical guideline). London: RCOG.

NHS Litigation Authority. (2009). *Clinical negligence scheme for trusts. Clinical risk management standards for the maternity services.* London: NHS Litigation Authority.

Westgate, J. A., Wibbens, B., & Bennet, L., et al. (2007). The intrapartum deceleration in center stage: a physiologic approach to the interpretation of fetal heart rate changes in labor. *American Journal of Obstetrics and Gynecology, 197,* 63–74.

Index

Note: Page numbers in italics refer to figures and tables.